Wall Pilates Workouts for Women

Transform Your Body in Just 21 Days with More than 175 STEP-BY-STEP VIDEOS and Illustrations. The 10-Minute Daily Guide to Toning.

Salena Hicks

Copyright © 2024 by Salena Hicks

All rights reserved.

No part of this publication may be reproduced, stored in a retrieval system, or transmitted in any form or by any means, electronic, mechanical, photocopying, recording, or otherwise, without the prior written permission of the publisher.

This publication is for personal use only.

Table of Contents

INTRODUCTION 5

CHAPTER 1: GETTING STARTED 7
    How to Download Your Bonuses 7
    Benefits of Wall Pilates 8
    Equipment and Setup 9
    Understanding and Preventing Injuries 10

CHAPTER 2: EXERCISES 12
    1. Wall Plank 12
    2. Wall Squats 14
    3. Wall Push-Ups 16
    4. Wall Sit with Leg Lifts 18
    5. Wall Bridge 20
    6. Wall Mountain Climbers 22
    7. Legs Up the Wall 24
    8. Wall Sit 26
    9. Seated Side Bends 28
    10. Wall Handstands 30
    11. Wall Shoulder Taps 32
    12. Wall Calf Raises 34
    13. Wall Side Plank 36
    14. Wall Diamond Push-Up 38
    15. Wall Hamstring Stretches 40
    16. Wall Triceps Push-Up 42
    17. Wall Donkey Kicks 44
    18. Wall Push-Ups with Leg Lifts 46
    19. Wall Bicycle Crunches 48
    20. Wall Side Leg Lifts 50
    21. Wall Crunches 52
    22. Wall Russian Twists 54
    23. Wall Arm Circles 56
    24. Wall Angel 58
    25. Standing Glute Kickbacks 60
    26. Wall Figure 4 Stretch 62
    27. Standing Leg Circles 64
    28. Wall Dead Bug 66

29. Wall Hip Flexor Stretches 68
30. Standing Wall Twist 70
31. Wall Side Lunges 72
32. Wall Walks 74
33. Wall Sprints (high knees against the wall) 76
34. Wall Splits 78
35. Wall Tricep Stretch 80
36. Wall Squats level 2 82
37. Wall Lateral Leg Swings 84
38. Wall Side Stretch 86
39. Wall Marches 88
40. The Spine Stretch 92
41. Wall Frog Stretch 94
42. Wall Pec Stretch 96
43. The Control Balance 98
44. Downward Facing Dog 100
45. Wall Wrist Stretches 104
46. Wall Butterfly Stretch 106
47. High Lunge Pose 110
48. Wall Roll Downs 112
49. Warrior 3 Pose 114
50. Half Plough Pose 116

CHAPTER 3: 21-DAY TRANSFORMATION CHALLENGE 118
Introduction to the 21-Day Challenge 118
Daily Schedule and Workout Plan 119

CHAPTER 4: NUTRITION AND WELLNESS 122
21-Day Meal Plan 122
Mindfulness and Holistic Well-being 125

CONCLUSION 127

Introduction

Welcome to "Wall Pilates Workouts for Women: Transform Your Body in Just 21 Days!" This comprehensive guide is designed to help you embark on a transformative journey towards a stronger, more toned physique using the innovative approach of Wall Pilates.

In today's fast-paced world, finding an effective and convenient workout routine is essential. This book is your gateway to an empowering fitness regimen that harnesses the support of a simple yet versatile tool—the wall. With over 50 carefully curated exercises and a structured 21-day challenge, this guide provides you with the tools and techniques needed to revitalize your fitness journey. And more in the bonuses section.

What You'll Discover:
Step-by-Step Guidance: Clear instructions and illustrations accompany each exercise, ensuring proper form and technique.

Efficient Workouts: Experience the power of 10-minute daily workouts designed to target and tone key muscle groups.

Comprehensive 21-Day Challenge: A transformative journey awaits you, carefully structured to challenge and progress with each passing day.

Inclusivity and Adaptability: Whether you're a beginner or a fitness enthusiast, these workouts are adaptable to various fitness levels and can be performed at your own pace.

Why Wall Pilates?
Wall Pilates offers a unique fusion of traditional Pilates principles with the added stability and support of the wall. This integration amplifies the effectiveness of each movement, allowing for better alignment, increased muscle engagement, and reduced risk of injury.

How to Use This Book:

Before diving into the workouts, take advantage of the introductory sections covering topics such as how to download your bonuses, guidance on utilizing this book effectively, and important insights on injury prevention and management. These sections will set the stage for a successful and fulfilling fitness journey.

Are you ready to embrace the transformative power of Wall Pilates and embark on a 21-day journey to a stronger, more toned you? Let's begin this empowering adventure together!

Chapter 1: Getting Started

How to Download Your Bonuses

Unlock Your Exclusive Bonuses!

Congratulations on purchasing "Wall Pilates Workouts for Women"! As a token of our appreciation, we're thrilled to offer you exclusive bonuses to complement your fitness journey.

To access your bonuses, follow these simple steps:

1. Scan the QR Code Below: Use your smartphone or tablet to scan the QR code provided. This will take you to a page where you can enter your email address.

2. Enter Your Email Address: Once you've scanned the QR code, enter your email address in the designated field.

3. Receive Your Bonus Email: After submitting your email address, you'll receive an email containing links to download all the bonuses. Check your inbox (and spam folder, just in case) for the email titled "Your Exclusive Bonuses Await!"

4. Download Your Bonuses: Open the email and click on the provided link for every bonus to download it. You'll find everything you need to enhance your Pilates practice, including the fitness journal, smoothie recipes, motivational music playlist, bonus exercises with videos, and more!

We hope you enjoy these valuable resources and that they enhance your Pilates experience. Thank you for choosing "Wall Pilates Workouts for Women" to support your fitness journey!

In case you don't receive your bonuses please send a message to pilates@salenahicks.online

Benefits of Wall Pilates

Enhanced Stability and Support: The wall acts as a stable surface, providing support for various movements, aiding balance, and allowing practitioners to focus on refining their form without worrying about instability.

Improved Alignment and Posture: The wall serves as a point of reference, encouraging proper alignment during exercises. This helps in correcting posture issues and reducing strain on the spine, leading to better overall posture and spinal health.

Increased Muscle Engagement: Utilizing the wall adds resistance to movements, engaging muscles more deeply and effectively. This increased engagement amplifies the effectiveness of exercises, leading to better muscle toning and strengthening.

Greater Range of Motion: The support from the wall enables practitioners to explore a wider range of motion in certain exercises, facilitating better flexibility and mobility in joints and muscles.

Reduced Risk of Injury: With the focus on proper alignment and support, Wall Pilates can minimize the risk of injury by promoting controlled movements and reducing strain on vulnerable areas of the body.

Core Strengthening: Like traditional Pilates, Wall Pilates emphasizes core strength. The integration of the wall further challenges the core muscles, fostering a stronger and more stable core.

Versatility and Adaptability: Wall Pilates exercises can be modified and adapted to accommodate different fitness levels and abilities, making them accessible to a wide range of individuals.

Mind-Body Connection: Practicing Wall Pilates encourages mindfulness, as it requires focus on breath, movement, and alignment. This fosters a deeper mind-body connection, promoting mental relaxation and stress relief.

Holistic Fitness: Beyond physical benefits, Wall Pilates contributes to overall well-being by enhancing balance, coordination, and body awareness, thus promoting a sense of overall fitness and wellness.

These benefits collectively make Wall Pilates an appealing and effective exercise approach, offering a holistic way to enhance strength, flexibility, and mental focus while prioritizing safe and controlled movements.

Equipment and Setup

The beauty of Wall Pilates lies in its simplicity and minimal equipment requirements. Here's an overview of the equipment and setup needed for Wall Pilates workouts:

Equipment:
Wall: A sturdy and clear wall space is the primary requirement. Ensure the wall is free from obstacles or distractions to allow for a safe and uninterrupted workout experience.

Yoga Mat or Exercise Mat: While not mandatory, a mat can provide cushioning and comfort, especially for floor-based exercises or stretches.

Setup:
Clear Space: Choose a wall with ample space around it to comfortably perform exercises without obstruction.

Positioning: Stand or sit with your back against the wall, maintaining proper posture. Ensure there's enough space to move arms and legs freely during exercises without hitting nearby furniture or objects.

Mat Placement: If using a mat, place it on the floor in front of the wall, allowing enough room for movements and stretches.

Optional Equipment:
Although Wall Pilates primarily relies on the wall for support, here are a few optional items that might enhance the workout experience:

Resistance Bands: Adding resistance bands can amplify the challenge and engage muscles further in certain exercises.

Small Stability Ball: Some exercises can incorporate a small stability ball against the wall to increase intensity and target specific muscle groups.

Yoga Blocks: These can aid in certain stretches or modifications, providing additional support or extension for some movements.

Safety Precautions:

Before starting any exercise regimen, ensure the wall is clean, dry, and free from any hazards.

Use caution when performing exercises, especially if you have any pre-existing health conditions or injuries. Always prioritize proper form and technique to prevent injury.

By keeping the setup simple and utilizing the support of a wall, Wall Pilates offers a convenient and effective way to engage in a full-body workout regimen from the comfort of your home or any suitable space. Adjustments and modifications can always be made to suit individual preferences and fitness levels.

Understanding and Preventing Injuries

In any fitness journey, understanding how to prevent injuries is as important as achieving fitness goals. Wall Pilates workouts offer incredible benefits, but ensuring safety and injury prevention is paramount to a successful and sustainable practice.

Understanding Common Injuries:

Strains and Sprains: Overexertion or improper technique can lead to strains in muscles or ligament sprains.

Joint Pain: Incorrect alignment or excessive stress on joints can lead to discomfort or pain in areas like the knees, hips, or shoulders.

Lower Back Issues: Improper form or excessive arching can cause lower back strain or discomfort.

Preventing Injuries in Wall Pilates:

Proper Form and Technique: Focus on correct posture and alignment in each exercise, engaging core muscles to support movements.

Gradual Progression: Avoid pushing beyond your limits too quickly; gradually increase intensity and difficulty over time.

Listen to Your Body: Pay attention to any discomfort or pain. If something doesn't feel right, modify the exercise or consult a professional.

Warm-up and Cool-down: Prioritize warming up before workouts and cooling down afterward to prepare your muscles and aid recovery.

Rest and Recovery: Allow your body sufficient rest between sessions to prevent overtraining and give your muscles time to recover.

Always watch the videos:

Consider watching the video first and then performing the exercise. Every single exercise in the book has its own unique video in the bonuses section, so use it to your advantage. They can provide guidance on proper techniques and personalized modifications to suit your body's needs.

Adapting to Individual Needs:

Everybody is different. Respect your body's limitations and adapt exercises as needed. Modify movements to accommodate any injuries, limitations, or discomfort.

Conclusion: Prioritize Safety and Longevity

Understanding potential risks and implementing injury prevention strategies are crucial for a safe and sustainable Wall Pilates practice. By prioritizing proper form, gradual progression, and listening to your body, you not only minimize injury risks but also promote a more fulfilling and enjoyable fitness journey.

Don't forget, the goal is not just immediate progress but long-term well-being. Prioritize safety, be mindful of your body's signals, and embark on your Wall Pilates journey with a commitment to injury prevention for a sustainable and rewarding practice.

Chapter 2: Exercises

1. Wall Plank

How to do a Wall Plank:

1. Positioning: Stand facing the wall, about an arm's length away. Place your hands flat on the wall, slightly wider than shoulder-width apart, at shoulder height or slightly higher.

2. Alignment: Extend your arms fully, ensuring they're parallel to the floor. Your body should form a straight line from head to heels, with your feet hip-width apart and flat on the floor.

3. Engage Core Muscles: Engage your abdominal muscles by drawing your navel towards your spine. This helps maintain stability and support for your lower back.

4. Lean Forward: Slowly lean your body weight forward by pressing into the wall with your hands, keeping your arms straight. Maintain a strong core and avoid arching your back excessively.

5. Hold the Plank: Hold this position for a set duration, such as 20-30 seconds for beginners, gradually increasing the time as you gain strength and endurance. Focus on breathing steadily throughout the exercise.

6. Exit the Plank: To release, gently push away from the wall and return to a standing position.

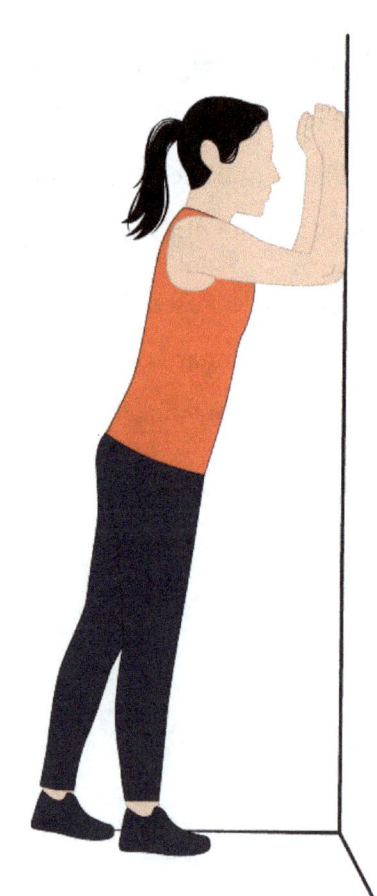

Tips for Performing Wall Planks:

- Focus on maintaining a neutral spine throughout the exercise to avoid overarching or rounding of the back.

- Keep your neck in line with your spine by looking at the wall or slightly downwards.

- Ensure your shoulders are relaxed, away from your ears, to prevent tension buildup.

Benefits of Wall Planks:

- Strengthens the core muscles, including the abdominals and lower back.

- Improves shoulder stability and arm strength.

- Enhances overall posture by engaging and stabilizing the muscles along the spine.

2. Wall Squats

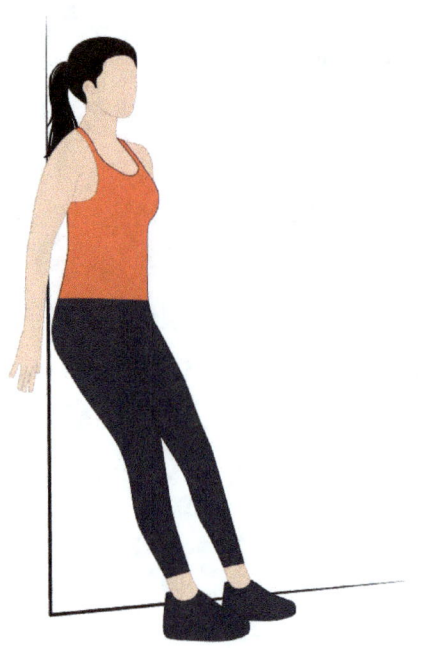
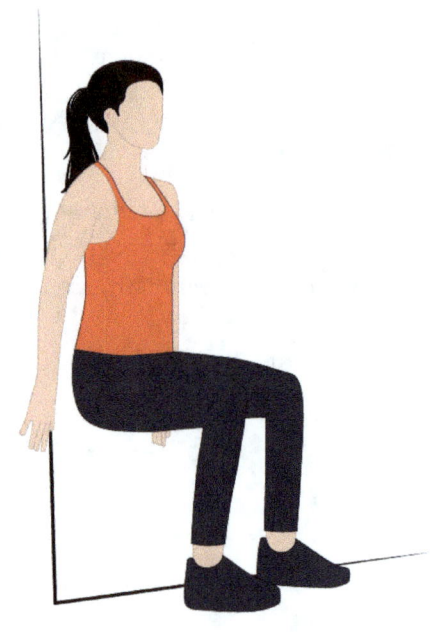

How to do Wall Squats:

1. Positioning: Stand with your back against the wall and your feet hip-width apart, about a foot away from the wall. Your feet should be flat on the floor, and your lower back and shoulders should be in contact with the wall.

2. Engage Core Muscles: Engage your abdominal muscles by drawing your navel towards your spine. Maintain this engagement throughout the exercise to support your lower back.

3. Initiate the Squat: Slowly slide your back down the wall while bending your knees, as if you're sitting into an imaginary chair. Lower your body until your thighs are parallel to the floor or as close to parallel as comfortable, keeping your knees aligned with your ankles and not extending beyond your toes.

4. Alignment: Ensure your back stays against the wall throughout the movement, and your heels remain flat on the floor. Your knees should be in line with your toes, not caving inward.

5. Hold the Squat: Hold this position for a set duration, such as 20-30 seconds for beginners. Focus on breathing steadily and maintaining proper form.

6. Return to Standing: Push through your heels and engage your leg muscles to slowly slide back up the wall to the starting position without using your hands for support.

Tips for Performing Wall Squats:

- Keep your chest lifted and your gaze straight ahead to maintain proper alignment of your spine.

- Avoid letting your knees extend beyond your toes to prevent excessive strain on the knee joints.

- Focus on pressing through your heels as you rise from the squat position to engage the glutes and hamstrings effectively.

Benefits of Wall Squats:

- Strengthens the muscles of the lower body, including the quadriceps, hamstrings, and glutes.

- Helps improve overall lower body endurance and stability.

- Provides a low-impact exercise option that's gentle on the knees while still being effective for building lower body strength.

3. Wall Push-Ups

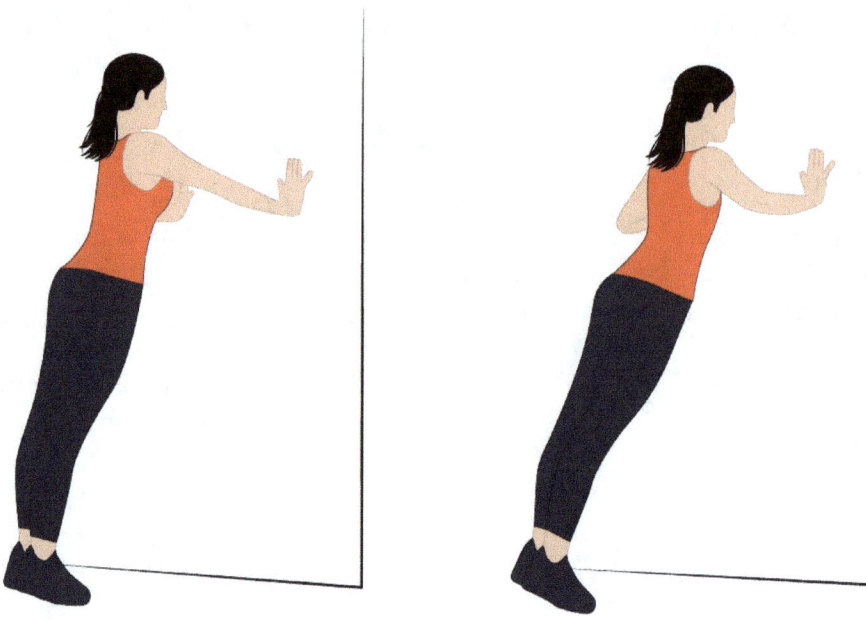

How to do Wall Push-Ups:

1. Positioning: Stand facing the wall, approximately arm's length away. Place your palms flat on the wall at shoulder height or slightly wider than shoulder-width apart, with your arms extended.

2. Alignment: Keep your body in a straight line from head to heels, engaging your core muscles to maintain stability. Your feet should be hip-width apart and flat on the floor.

3. Engage Core Muscles: Draw your navel towards your spine to engage your abdominal muscles. This helps maintain proper alignment and support for your lower back.

4. Bend Your Arms: Slowly bend your elbows and lower your chest towards the wall while maintaining a straight body position. Keep your elbows close to your body as you lower yourself.

5. Push Back Up: Push through your palms and straighten your arms to return to the starting position, extending your elbows fully without locking them.

6. Breathing: Exhale as you push away from the wall and inhale as you lower your chest towards the wall.

Tips for Performing Wall Push-Ups:

- Ensure your body remains in a straight line throughout the exercise, avoiding arching or sagging of the back.

- Focus on the movement coming from your arms and chest muscles, keeping the core engaged for stability.

- Keep your neck in line with your spine, looking at the wall to maintain proper alignment.

Benefits of Wall Push-Ups:

- Strengthens the muscles of the chest, shoulders, arms, and core.

- Offers a beginner-friendly variation of the traditional push-up, allowing individuals to build upper body strength gradually.

- Can be performed anywhere with a wall, making it a convenient exercise for home workouts or while traveling.

4. Wall Sit with Leg Lifts

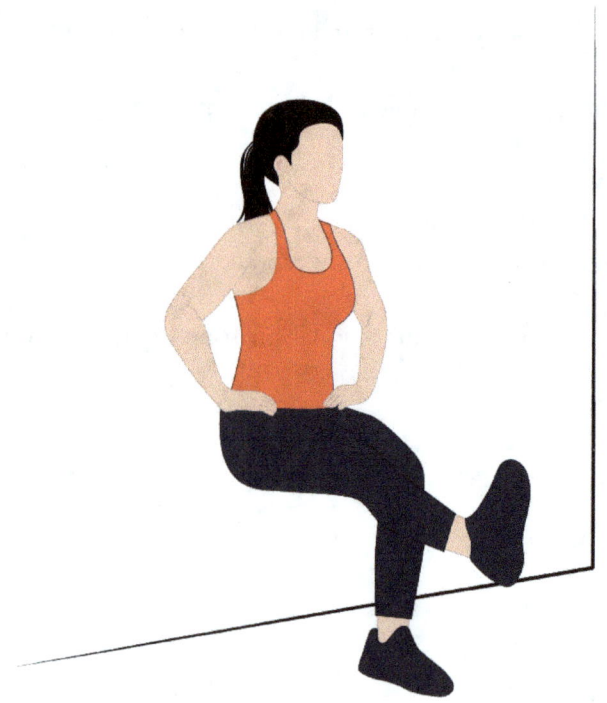

How to do Wall Sit with Leg Lifts:

1. Positioning: Stand with your back against the wall and your feet hip-width apart, about 2 feet away from the wall. Slide down the wall until your knees are bent at a 90-degree angle, as if sitting in an imaginary chair. Ensure your lower back and shoulders are in contact with the wall.

2. Engage Core Muscles: Engage your abdominal muscles by drawing your navel towards your spine. Maintain this engagement throughout the exercise to support your lower back.

3. Wall Sit: Hold the wall sit position with your thighs parallel to the floor or as close to parallel as comfortable. Your knees should be aligned with your ankles, and your weight should be evenly distributed on both feet.

4. Leg Lifts: While maintaining the wall sit position, lift one leg straight out in front of you, keeping it parallel to the floor for a few seconds. Lower it back down and repeat with the other leg.

5. Alternate Leg Lifts: Continue alternating leg lifts, ensuring controlled movements and maintaining the wall sit position throughout.

6. Breathing: Breathe steadily throughout the exercise, exhaling as you lift your leg and inhaling as you lower it back down.

Tips for Performing Wall Sit with Leg Lifts:

- Keep your back flat against the wall and avoid arching or rounding your back.

- Focus on engaging your core muscles to stabilize your body during leg lifts.

- Keep both knees and toes pointed forward throughout the exercise.

Benefits of Wall Sit with Leg Lifts:

- Strengthens the quadriceps, hamstrings, glutes, and core muscles.

- Challenges stability and balance while targeting multiple lower body muscle groups simultaneously.

- Can be modified to suit different fitness levels by adjusting the duration of the wall sit or the height of leg lifts.

5. Wall Bridge

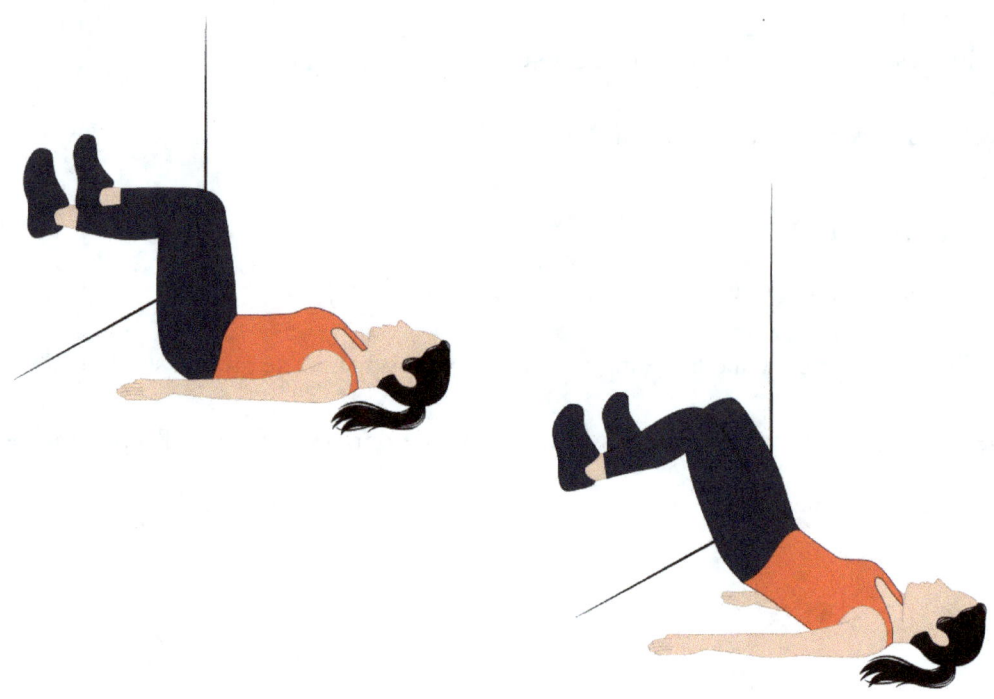

How to do Wall Bridge:

1. Positioning: Lie on your back with your feet flat on the floor, knees bent at approximately a 90-degree angle, and arms by your sides. Ensure your heels are about a foot away from the wall.

2. Engage Core Muscles: Engage your abdominal muscles by gently drawing your navel towards your spine. This helps maintain stability and support for your lower back.

3. Initiate the Bridge: Press your feet firmly into the floor and lift your hips towards the ceiling, driving through your heels. Simultaneously, slide your feet up the wall, straightening your legs as much as comfortable.

4. Form the Bridge: Aim to create a straight line from your shoulders to your knees while keeping your shoulders, upper back, and head on the floor. You'll feel a contraction in your glutes and hamstrings.

5. Hold the Bridge: Hold this position for a few seconds, focusing on squeezing your glutes and maintaining stability. Ensure your core remains engaged throughout the movement.

6. Lower Down: Slowly lower your hips back down to the floor, returning to the starting position with control.

Tips for Performing Wall Bridge:

- Avoid arching your lower back excessively during the bridge; aim to maintain a neutral spine.

- Keep your neck relaxed and avoid straining it by looking straight ahead or towards the ceiling.

- Focus on breathing steadily throughout the exercise, inhaling as you prepare and exhaling as you lift into the bridge.

Benefits of Wall Bridge:

- Strengthens the glutes, hamstrings, and lower back muscles.

- Improves hip stability, flexibility, and mobility.

- Engages the core muscles for stability and balance.

6. Wall Mountain Climbers

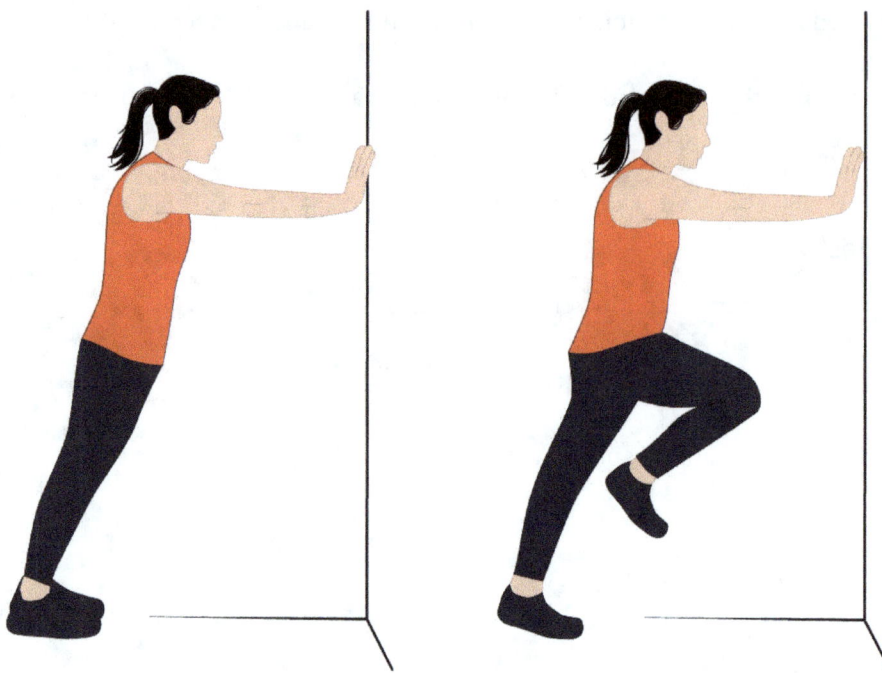

How to do Wall Mountain Climbers:

1. Find a Wall: Stand facing a sturdy wall with enough space around you to move your legs freely.

2. Assume the Starting Position: Stand up straight with your feet shoulder-width apart and your arms extended in front of you, palms flat against the wall at shoulder height. Your body should form a straight line from head to heels.

3. Engage Your Core: Tighten your abdominal muscles to stabilize your torso.

4. Begin the Movement: In a controlled manner, lift your right knee towards your chest while simultaneously pulling your left arm back, as if you were running in place. Your left knee should remain extended as your right knee drives up.

5. Switch Legs and Arms: As you lower your right leg back down, immediately lift your left knee towards your chest while pulling your right arm back. It's important to maintain a fluid motion, alternating between legs and arms.

6. Maintain a Quick Pace: Aim for a brisk, rhythmic pace to keep your heart rate elevated and maximize the cardiovascular benefits of the exercise.

7. Focus on Form: Keep your back straight, shoulders down and relaxed, and core engaged throughout the movement. Avoid leaning too far forward or backward.

8. Repeat: Continue alternating between legs and arms for the desired number of repetitions or time duration.

9. Cool Down: Once you've completed your set, take a few moments to stretch your muscles, focusing on the calves, hamstrings, quadriceps, and shoulders.

Tips for Performing Wall Mountain Climbers:

- Focus on driving your knees towards your chest with control and precision rather than speed.

- Keep your shoulders directly above your wrists and your core engaged to stabilize your body.

- Maintain a steady and controlled breathing pattern throughout the exercise.

Benefits of Wall Mountain Climbers:

- Engages and strengthens the core muscles, including the abdominals, obliques, and lower back.

- Targets the shoulders, arms, and chest muscles, promoting upper body strength and stability.

- Provides a cardiovascular challenge while enhancing coordination and agility.

7. Legs Up the Wall

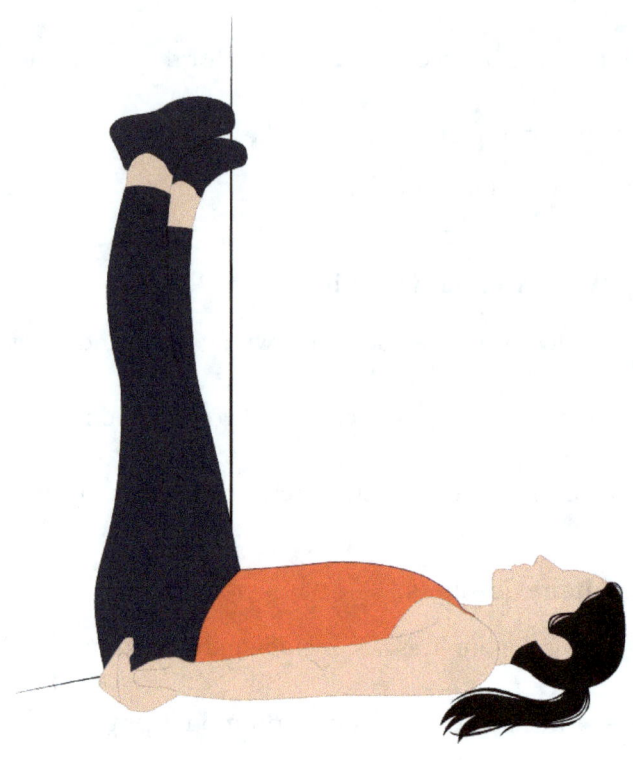

How to do Legs Up the Wall:

1. Preparation: Find an open wall space, preferably free from obstacles. Sit close to the wall sideways, with one hip against the wall.

2. Positioning: Gently lie down on your back while simultaneously swinging your legs up against the wall. Your hips should be as close to the wall as is comfortable, and your legs extended upward along the wall.

3. Adjustment: If needed, shift your body or move away from the wall slightly to find a position where your legs feel relaxed without any strain or discomfort. Your back should be comfortable on the floor.

4. Arms Position: Extend your arms comfortably by your sides or rest them on your abdomen or chest. Relax your shoulders and let them rest comfortably on the ground.

5. Breathing and Relaxation: Close your eyes and focus on your breath. Take slow, deep breaths, allowing your body to relax and your mind to unwind. Remain in this position for 5-15 minutes, or as long as desired.

6. Exiting the Pose: To release, gently bend your knees and roll to one side before slowly rising to a seated position.

Tips for Legs Up the Wall:

- Use a folded blanket or cushion under your hips or lower back for added support and comfort if needed.

- Keep the neck and head in a neutral position, ensuring there's no strain or tension in the neck.

- Engage in deep, mindful breathing to encourage relaxation and release tension.

Benefits of Legs Up the Wall:

- Improves Circulation: This pose allows for enhanced blood flow from the legs back towards the heart, which can reduce swelling and alleviate tiredness in the legs.

- Relaxation and Stress Relief: Legs Up the Wall is known for its calming effects, promoting relaxation and reducing stress and anxiety.

- Soothing for the Nervous System: This pose encourages the body's parasympathetic nervous system, aiding in relaxation and promoting a sense of calm.

8. Wall Sit

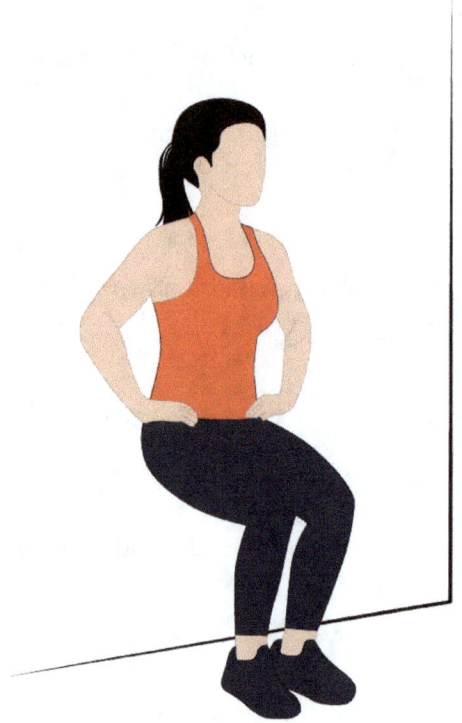

How to do a Wall Sit:

1. Positioning: Stand with your back against a wall and your feet positioned about shoulder-width apart, approximately 1 to 2 feet away from the wall.

2. Lowering into the Wall Sit: Slowly slide your back down the wall, bending your knees until they're at a 90-degree angle or as close to a right angle as is comfortable. Aim to have your thighs parallel to the floor.

3. Alignment: Ensure your lower back and entire spine remain in contact with the wall throughout the exercise. Your feet should be flat on the ground, and your knees should be directly above your ankles, not extending beyond your toes.

4. Form Check: Check to ensure your weight is evenly distributed between both feet, and your heels are bearing a significant portion of the load to engage the glutes and hamstrings effectively.

5. Hold the Wall Sit: Hold this position for a set duration, such as 20-60 seconds for beginners or longer for those more experienced. Focus on breathing steadily throughout the hold.

6. Rising from the Wall Sit: Push through your heels and engage your leg muscles to slowly slide back up the wall to the starting position. Avoid using momentum or bouncing to rise.

Tips for Performing a Wall Sit:

- Keep your core engaged by drawing your navel towards your spine to support your lower back.

- Ensure your knees are aligned with your toes and do not cave inward or extend beyond your toes to prevent excess strain on the knees.

- Focus on maintaining a neutral spine and avoiding arching or rounding of the lower back.

Benefits of Wall Sits:

- Strengthens the muscles of the lower body, including the quadriceps, hamstrings, glutes, and calves.

- Improves muscular endurance and stability in the lower body.

- Provides a low-impact exercise option that doesn't require additional equipment.

9. Seated Side Bends

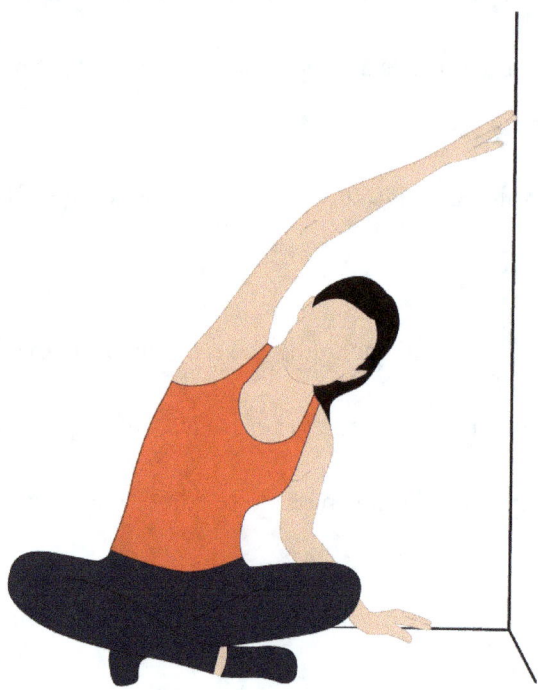

How to do Seated Side Bends:

1. Find a Comfortable Seated Position: Sit on the floor or on a mat with your legs extended in front of you.

2. Cross Your Legs: Cross your legs at the ankles or bring one foot over the other, placing the ankle on top of the opposite knee. Choose a comfortable position that allows you to maintain balance and stability throughout the exercise.

3. Engage Your Core: Sit up tall with your spine straight and shoulders relaxed. Engage your abdominal muscles to stabilize your torso.

4. Position Your Arms: Extend your arms out to the sides, parallel to the floor, with your palms facing down. This will help you maintain balance and stability during the movement.

5. Perform the Side Bend: Inhale as you lengthen through your spine, and then exhale as you lean to one side, bringing your hand towards the floor. Keep your chest open and facing forward, and avoid collapsing your torso forward or rounding your back.

6. Feel the Stretch: You should feel a stretch along the side of your torso on the opposite side of the bend.

7. Return to Center: Inhale as you come back to the starting position, engaging your core to lift yourself back up to an upright position.

8. Repeat on the Other Side: Exhale as you perform a side bend to the opposite side, maintaining the crossed-leg position. Keep your movements controlled and deliberate.

9. Continue Alternating Sides: Repeat the side bends for the desired number of repetitions or time duration, alternating sides with each repetition.

10. Focus on Breathing: Remember to coordinate your breath with your movements, inhaling as you lengthen through your spine and exhaling as you perform the side bend.

11. Cool Down: Once you've completed your set, take a few moments to stretch your side body and lower back to help release any tension.

Tips for Seated Side Bends:

- Keep both buttocks firmly planted on the floor throughout the movement to isolate the stretch to the sides of the torso.

- Avoid collapsing or rounding your back; aim to maintain a tall, extended spine during the side bends.

- Perform the movement slowly and smoothly, focusing on the stretch and breathing rhythmically.

Benefits of Seated Side Bends:

- Oblique Strengthening: Targets and strengthens the oblique muscles along the sides of the torso.

- Spinal Mobility: Promotes flexibility and mobility in the spine, particularly in lateral (side-to-side) movements.

- Improved Posture: Enhances awareness of posture and encourages a taller, more elongated spine.

10. Wall Handstands

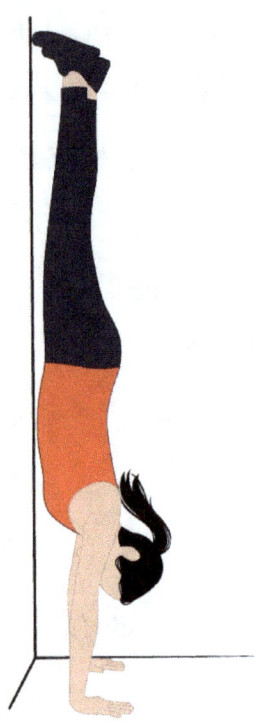

How to do Wall Handstands:

1. Preparation: Find an open space near a wall. Place a mat or cushioned surface against the wall to support your back and head.

2. Starting Position: Begin in a kneeling position facing away from the wall. Place your hands on the floor shoulder-width apart, approximately 6-12 inches away from the wall.

3. Positioning the Body: Slowly lift your hips and straighten your legs, walking your feet closer to your hands until your body forms an inverted "V" shape with your hips over your shoulders. This is the starting position.

4. Kicking Up: With control, lift one leg off the ground and use the other foot to push against the floor, aiming to kick up gently while the wall provides support. As you gain confidence, aim to kick up both legs simultaneously, transitioning into a handstand position.

5. Aligning Against the Wall: Once in the handstand position, position your back against the wall, allowing your feet to rest on the wall for support. Your body should form a straight line from wrists to shoulders, hips, and heels.

6. Balance and Engagement: Engage your core muscles, press through your palms, and focus on maintaining a stable, straight body position. Keep your gaze focused between your hands to assist with balance.

7. Hold and Breathe: Hold the handstand position for a comfortable duration, aiming to maintain balance and control. Breathe deeply and evenly throughout the hold.

8. Exiting the Handstand: Lower your legs back to the starting "V" position by gently bending your knees and controlling your descent.

Tips for Wall Handstands:

- Practice near a soft surface or use a spotter when learning to ensure safety.

- Start with shorter holds and gradually increase the duration as strength and confidence improve.

- Use the wall for support and to familiarize yourself with the inverted position before attempting to balance without it.

Benefits of Wall Handstands:

- Strength Building: Engages the upper body, including shoulders, arms, and core muscles.

- Improved Balance and Body Awareness: Enhances proprioception and balance by challenging spatial awareness.

- Increased Confidence: Progressing in handstands can boost confidence and body control.

11. Wall Shoulder Taps

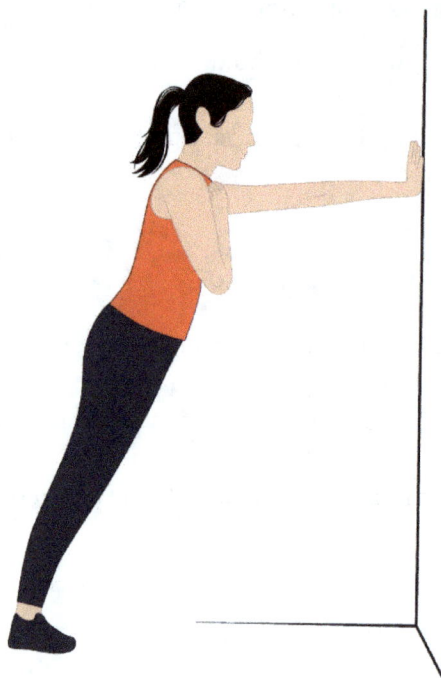

How to do Wall Shoulder Taps:

1. Find a Wall: Stand facing a sturdy wall with enough space around you to extend your arms and move your body.

2. Assume the Plank Position: Place your hands flat on the wall at about shoulder height, slightly wider than shoulder-width apart. Extend your arms fully and walk your feet back until your body forms a straight line from head to heels, similar to the plank position.

3. Engage Your Core: Tighten your abdominal muscles to stabilize your torso. Your body should be in a straight line, and your hips shouldn't be sagging or picking up.

4. Tap Your Shoulders: Once you're in a stable plank position, lift your right hand off the wall and tap your left shoulder with it. Keep your hips and torso as still as possible to avoid excessive rotation.

5. Alternate Sides: After tapping your left shoulder with your right hand, return your right hand to the starting position on the wall, then lift your left hand and tap your right shoulder with it. Continue alternating between tapping each shoulder.

6. Maintain Control: Focus on maintaining a stable plank position throughout the exercise. Avoid rocking or swaying your body as you tap your shoulders.

7. Control Your Breathing: Breathe steadily and rhythmically throughout the exercise. Inhale as you prepare to tap your shoulder, and exhale as you lift your hand and tap.

8. Keep Your Neck Neutral: Avoid straining your neck by keeping it in a neutral position, aligned with your spine. Look down at the floor slightly in front of your hands.

9. Perform for Repetitions or Time: You can perform standing wall shoulder taps for a certain number of repetitions (e.g., 10 taps per side) or for a set amount of time (e.g., 30 seconds to 1 minute).

10. Gradually Increase Difficulty: As you become more proficient at the exercise, you can increase the challenge by either extending the duration of each set or by placing your hands on a higher surface to decrease the angle of your body.

11. Cool Down: After completing your sets, stretch your shoulders, arms, and core to help relax the muscles and prevent tightness.

Tips for Wall Shoulder Taps:

- Keep your core engaged throughout the movement to stabilize your body and prevent excessive hip movement.

- Maintain a neutral spine and avoid rotating your hips; aim to keep your body in a straight line.

- Perform the movement slowly and with control to maximize the engagement of core muscles.

Benefits of Wall Shoulder Taps:

- Core Strengthening: Targets the core muscles, including the abdominals and obliques, while also engaging the shoulders and arms.

- Improved Stability: Enhances core stability, balance, and coordination.

- Variation in Plank Exercises: Offers a challenging variation of the traditional plank exercise by incorporating movement and coordination.

12. Wall Calf Raises

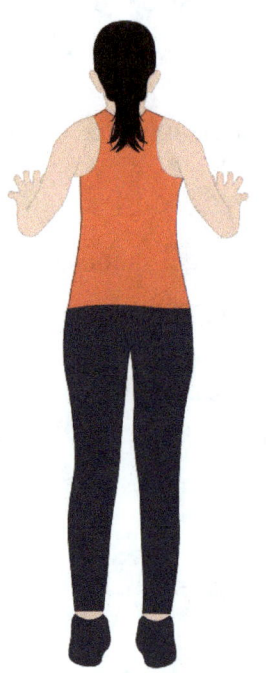 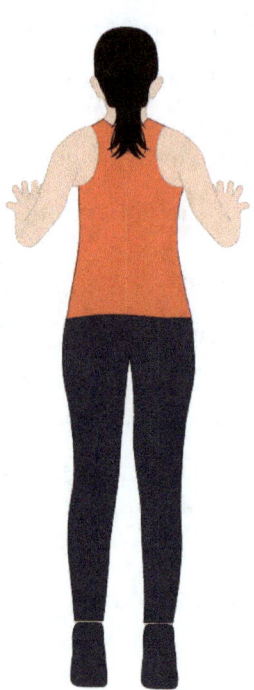

How to do Wall Calf Raises:

1. Positioning: Stand facing a wall, about an arm's length away, and place your palms flat against the wall at shoulder height for support. Your feet should be hip-width apart and flat on the ground.

2. Engage Core Muscles: Engage your core by drawing your navel toward your spine. This helps maintain stability throughout the exercise.

3. Performing the Calf Raise:

    o Slowly rise onto the balls of your feet, lifting your heels as high as comfortable while keeping your body straight.

    o Pause at the top of the movement, briefly holding the raised position to contract your calf muscles.

4. Lower Down: Gently lower your heels back to the starting position, allowing your heels to descend below the level of your toes to stretch the calf muscles.

5. Repetition: Repeat the movement for a set number of repetitions (e.g., 10-15 reps) or perform the exercise for a specific duration (e.g., 30 seconds).

6. Breathing: Exhale as you rise onto your toes and inhale as you lower your heels back down.

Tips for Wall Calf Raises:

- Focus on controlled movements throughout the exercise, avoiding rapid or jerky motions.

- Keep your body aligned and avoid leaning excessively forward or backward.

- Gradually increase the range of motion as your calf muscles become stronger and more flexible.

Benefits of Wall Calf Raises:

- Calf Muscle Strengthening: Targets and strengthens the calf muscles, particularly the gastrocnemius and soleus.

- Improved Ankle Stability: Enhances ankle strength and stability, which can be beneficial for activities involving running, jumping, and balance.

- Enhanced Lower Leg Definition: Regularly performing calf raises can help tone and define the lower leg muscles.

13. Wall Side Plank

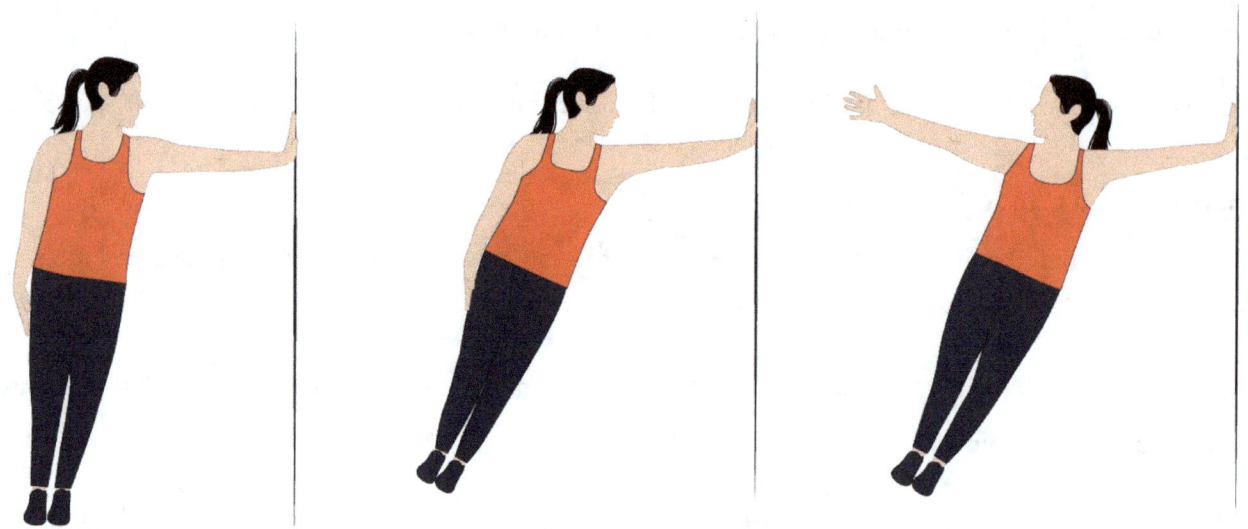

How to do Wall Side Plank:

1. Starting Position: Stand beside a wall, facing sideways. Place your forearm on the floor directly beneath your shoulder, parallel to the wall. Your elbow should be aligned with your shoulder, and your feet should be positioned against the wall.

2. Engage Core Muscles: Engage your core by drawing your navel toward your spine. This helps maintain stability throughout the exercise.

3. Lifting into the Side Plank:

   o Lift your hips off the ground, supporting your body weight on your forearm and the side of your bottom foot. Your body should form a straight line from head to heels.

   o Ensure your shoulders are stacked, one above the other, and your hips are lifted to prevent any sagging or tilting.

4. Alignment Check: Keep your body in a straight line without allowing your hips to drop towards the ground or pushing them too far upwards. Your head should be in line with your spine.

5. Hold the Plank: Hold the position for a set duration, such as 20-30 seconds for beginners, gradually increasing the time as you gain strength and endurance.

6. Repetition: Repeat the exercise on the opposite side by switching the position of your body, now facing the other direction.

Tips for Wall Side Plank:

- Focus on maintaining proper alignment and engaging the core muscles throughout the exercise.

- Keep your neck relaxed and in line with your spine, avoiding any strain or tension.

- Adjust the position of your feet against the wall to find a comfortable and stable stance.

Benefits of Wall Side Plank:

- Core Strengthening: Engages the obliques and deep core muscles for improved stability and strength.

- Shoulder and Hip Stability: Challenges shoulder and hip stability, promoting better overall body control.

- Variation in Core Exercises: Offers a dynamic variation of the side plank, adding a different challenge to the core muscles.

14. Wall Diamond Push-Up

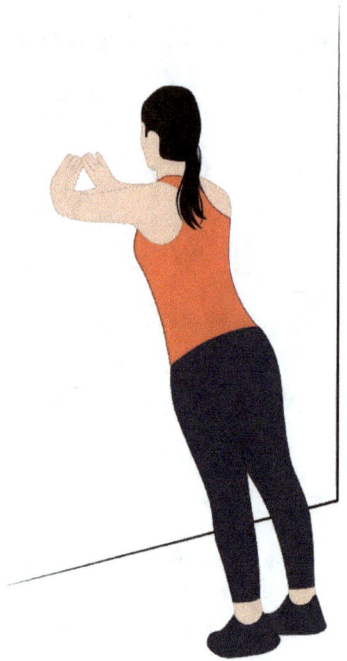

How to do Wall Diamond Push-Ups:

1. Positioning: Stand facing the wall and place your hands on the wall at shoulder-width apart, slightly closer than shoulder-width, forming a diamond shape with your thumbs and index fingers. Your hands should be at chest height or slightly higher.

2. Positioning the Body: Step back slightly from the wall, extending your arms so that your body forms a diagonal line from head to heels, leaning at an angle.

3. Engage Core Muscles: Engage your core by drawing your navel toward your spine. This helps maintain stability throughout the exercise.

4. Performing the Push-Up:

o Lower your chest towards the wall by bending your elbows, keeping them close to your body. Aim to bring your chest towards your hands while maintaining the diamond shape between them.

o Ensure a controlled descent, feeling the engagement in your triceps and chest muscles.

5. Push Back Up: Push through your palms, straightening your arms to return to the starting position without locking your elbows.

6. Repetition: Perform the desired number of repetitions, aiming for a set (e.g., 8-12 reps) or a specific duration.

Tips for Wall Diamond Push-Ups:

- Focus on maintaining proper form throughout the exercise, keeping your body in a straight line from head to heels.

- Control the movement both during the descent and ascent, avoiding rapid or jerky motions.

- Adjust the distance from the wall to increase or decrease the exercise difficulty.

Benefits of Wall Diamond Push-Ups:

- Triceps and Chest Strengthening: Targets the triceps (back of the arms) and chest muscles while engaging the shoulders.

- Modification for Beginners: Provides a modified variation for individuals unable to perform regular push-ups on the floor.

- Convenient and Accessible: Can be done almost anywhere with a wall, making it a convenient exercise option.

15. Wall Hamstring Stretches

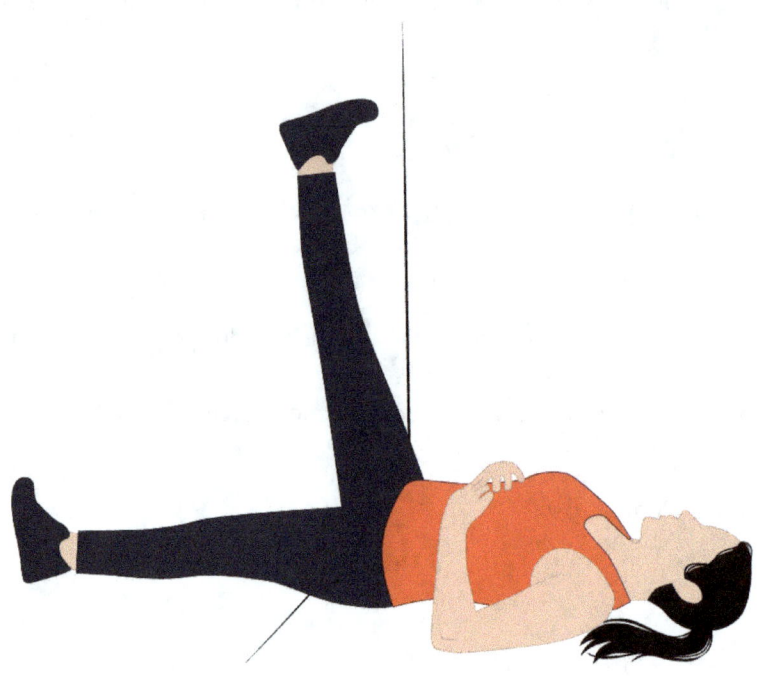

How to do Wall Hamstring Stretches:

1. Starting Position: Lie flat on your back near a wall, with your legs extended and your hips close to the wall.

2. Leg Positioning: Extend your legs up against the wall, resting your heels against the wall. Your body should form an L-shape, with your legs vertical and your torso flat on the ground.

3. Adjustment: If needed, move closer or farther from the wall to find a position where you feel a gentle stretch in your hamstrings without discomfort.

4. Relaxation: Allow your body to relax into the stretch, focusing on your breath. Take slow, deep breaths, allowing the muscles to gradually release and lengthen.

5. Hold the Stretch: Hold the position for 30 seconds to 2 minutes, depending on your comfort level and flexibility. Feel the stretch along the back of your thighs (hamstrings).

6. Exiting the Stretch: Gently bend your knees and slide your feet down the wall to return to the starting position.

- Modification : you can do it either by one leg at a time or both of them.

Tips for Wall Hamstring Stretches:

- Keep your legs relatively straight but avoid locking your knees to prevent strain.

- Engage in deep, relaxed breathing to encourage further relaxation and a deeper stretch.

- If you're unable to keep your legs fully extended against the wall, bend your knees slightly until you feel a comfortable stretch.

Benefits of Wall Hamstring Stretches:

- Improved Flexibility: Lengthens and relaxes the hamstring muscles, increasing flexibility.

- Reduced Tightness: Helps alleviate tightness in the hamstrings, which can benefit those with lower back discomfort or individuals who sit for long periods.

16. Wall Triceps Push-Up

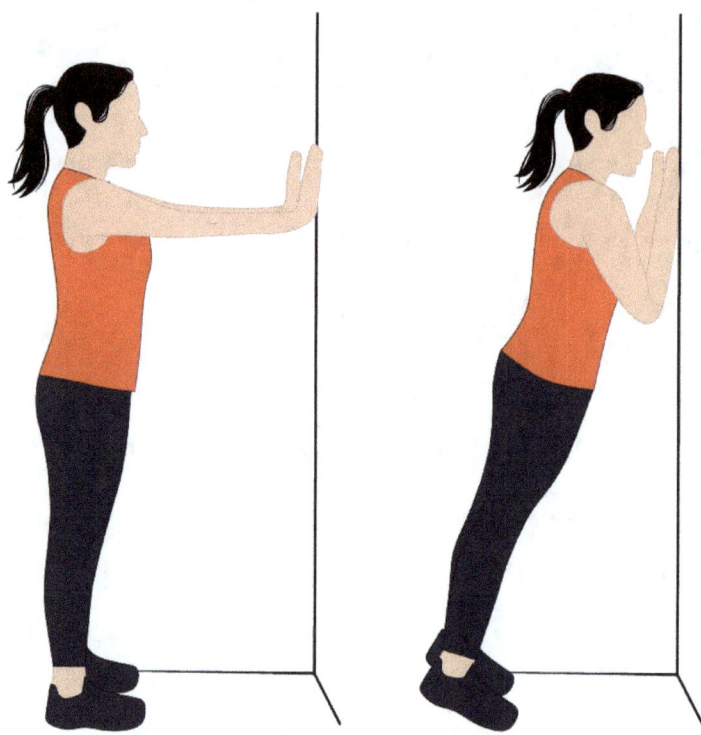

How to do Wall Triceps Push-Ups:

1. Positioning: Stand facing the wall and place your palms flat against the wall at shoulder-width apart, slightly lower than shoulder height. Your arms should be straight.

2. Positioning the Body: Step back slightly from the wall, extending your arms so that your body forms a diagonal line from head to heels, leaning at an angle.

3. Engage Core Muscles: Engage your core by drawing your navel toward your spine. This helps maintain stability throughout the exercise.

4. Performing the Push-Up:

    o Bend your elbows, lowering your chest toward the wall by leaning forward, keeping your elbows close to your body. Aim to bring your chest towards the wall while engaging your triceps.

    o Ensure a controlled descent, feeling the engagement in your triceps muscles.

5. Push Back Up: Push through your palms, straightening your arms to return to the starting position without locking your elbows.

6. Repetition: Perform the desired number of repetitions, aiming for a set (e.g., 8-12 reps) or a specific duration.

Tips for Wall Triceps Push-Ups:

- Focus on maintaining proper form throughout the exercise, keeping your body in a straight line from head to heels.

- Control the movement both during the descent and ascent, avoiding rapid or jerky motions.

- Adjust the distance from the wall to increase or decrease the exercise difficulty.

Benefits of Wall Triceps Push-Ups:

- Triceps Strengthening: Targets and strengthens the triceps (back of the arms) effectively.

- Accessible Exercise: Provides a modified variation for individuals who find regular push-ups challenging.

- Engagement of Upper Body Muscles: Engages the chest and shoulders to a lesser extent, offering a comprehensive upper body workout.

17. Wall Donkey Kicks

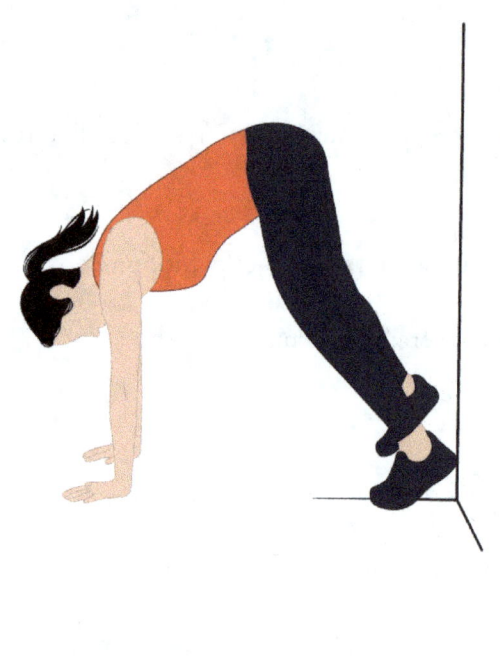
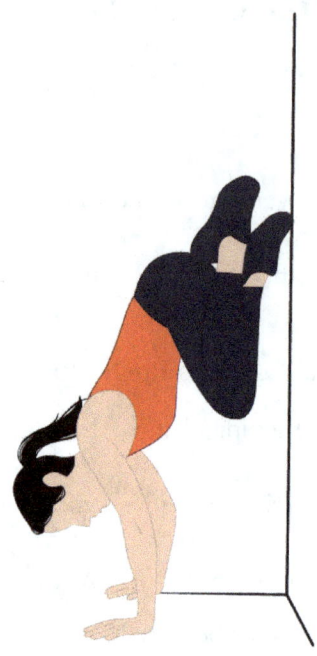

How to do Wall Donkey Kicks:

1. Starting Position: Begin by kneeling on all fours facing away from a wall. Place your hands shoulder-width apart on the floor and position your knees directly under your hips.

2. Positioning the Feet: Extend your legs and place your toes against the wall, pressing them firmly into the wall's surface. Your heels should be lifted off the ground.

3. Engage Core Muscles: Engage your core by drawing your navel toward your spine. This helps maintain stability throughout the exercise.

4. Performing the Donkey Kick:

    o Keeping your hands on the ground and your core engaged, simultaneously lift one leg up and back towards the ceiling in a kicking motion.

    o Aim to keep the knee bent at a 90-degree angle and the foot flexed as you push against the wall.

5. Squeeze and Lower: Pause at the top of the movement, squeezing your glutes, then slowly lower the leg back down without allowing it to touch the ground.

6. Alternate Legs: Repeat the movement with the other leg, performing an equal number of repetitions on each side.

Tips for Wall Donkey Kicks:

- Focus on maintaining control throughout the movement, avoiding any swinging or arching of the back.

- Keep your core engaged to stabilize your body and prevent excessive movement in the hips.

- Ensure that the movement comes from the glutes and hamstrings, not just the lower back.

Benefits of Wall Donkey Kicks:

- Glute and Hamstring Activation: Targets and strengthens the glutes and hamstrings effectively.

- Core Engagement: Engages the core muscles for stability and support during the movement.

- Convenient Variation: Offers a variation of the traditional donkey kicks using the support of a wall, making it convenient and effective.

18. Wall Push-Ups with Leg Lifts

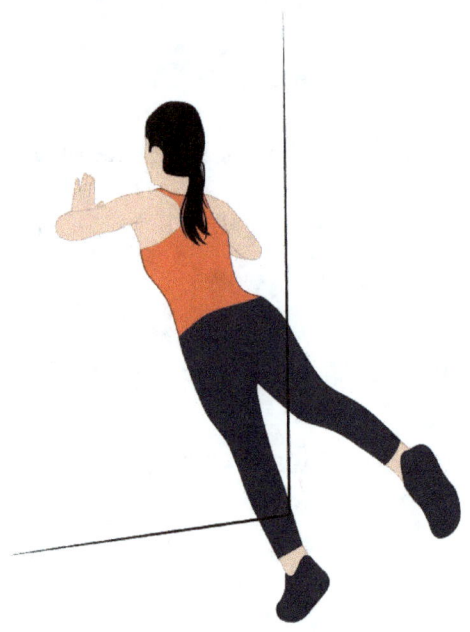

How to do Wall Push-Ups with Leg Lifts:

1. Starting Position: Stand facing the wall, about arm's length away. Place your palms flat against the wall at shoulder-width apart, slightly lower than shoulder height. Your arms should be straight.

2. Positioning the Body: Step back slightly from the wall, extending your arms so that your body forms a diagonal line from head to heels, leaning at an angle.

3. Engage Core Muscles: Engage your core by drawing your navel toward your spine. This helps maintain stability throughout the exercise.

4. Performing the Push-Up:

   o Perform a wall push-up by bending your elbows and lowering your chest towards the wall, keeping your body in a straight line.

   o As you push back to the starting position, simultaneously lift one leg off the ground, extending it backward.

5. Lower Leg and Repeat: Lower the lifted leg back to the ground while simultaneously performing another push-up, this time lifting the opposite leg.

6. Alternate Leg Lifts: Alternate lifting each leg with each push-up repetition, maintaining control and stability throughout the movement.

7. Repetition: Perform the desired number of push-ups with leg lifts, aiming for a set (e.g., 8-12 reps per leg) or a specific duration.

Tips for Wall Push-Ups with Leg Lifts:

- Focus on maintaining proper form throughout the exercise, keeping your body in a straight line from head to heels.

- Control the movement both during the push-up and leg lift, avoiding rapid or jerky motions.

- Engage the core muscles to stabilize the body as you lift each leg.

Benefits of Wall Push-Ups with Leg Lifts:

- Upper Body Strength: Targets the chest, shoulders, and arms with the push-up movement.

- Core and Lower Body Engagement: Engages the core, glutes, and lower body muscles with the leg lifts.

- Balance and Coordination: Challenges balance and coordination by incorporating leg lifts into the push-up movement.

19. Wall Bicycle Crunches

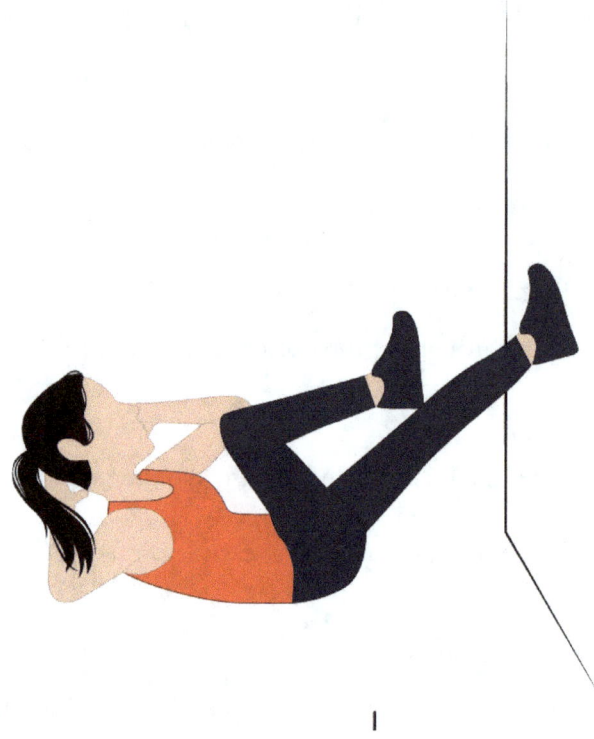

How to do Wall Bicycle Crunches:

1. Starting Position: Lie flat on your back on the floor or a mat with your hips close to the wall. Extend your legs upward, resting them against the wall. Your knees should be slightly bent.

2. Hand Positioning: Place your hands lightly behind your head, supporting your neck without pulling on it. Keep your elbows wide and avoid interlacing your fingers.

3. Engage Core Muscles: Engage your core by drawing your navel toward your spine. This helps maintain stability throughout the exercise.

4. Performing the Bicycle Crunch:

- Lift your head, neck, and shoulders slightly off the ground, gently pressing your lower back into the floor/mat.

- Simultaneously rotate your torso, bringing your right elbow towards your left knee while extending your right leg straight.

- Then switch, bringing your left elbow towards your right knee while extending your left leg straight. This mimics a cycling motion.

5. Breathing and Pace: Exhale as you crunch and rotate, inhale as you return to the starting position. Maintain a steady pace throughout the movement.

6. Repetition: Continue alternating the twisting motion, performing the exercise for a set number of repetitions or a specific duration.

Tips for Wall Bicycle Crunches:

- Focus on quality over quantity, ensuring controlled and deliberate movements throughout.

- Keep your lower back pressed against the floor/mat to engage the core effectively and prevent strain.

- Avoid pulling on your neck with your hands; instead, use them for light support.

Benefits of Wall Bicycle Crunches:

- Core Strengthening: Targets the rectus abdominis, obliques, and deeper core muscles effectively.

- Improved Flexibility and Stability: Enhances core flexibility and stability while engaging in a twisting motion.

- Accessible Variation: Offers a modified version of bicycle crunches that can be done against a wall for added support.

20. Wall Side Leg Lifts

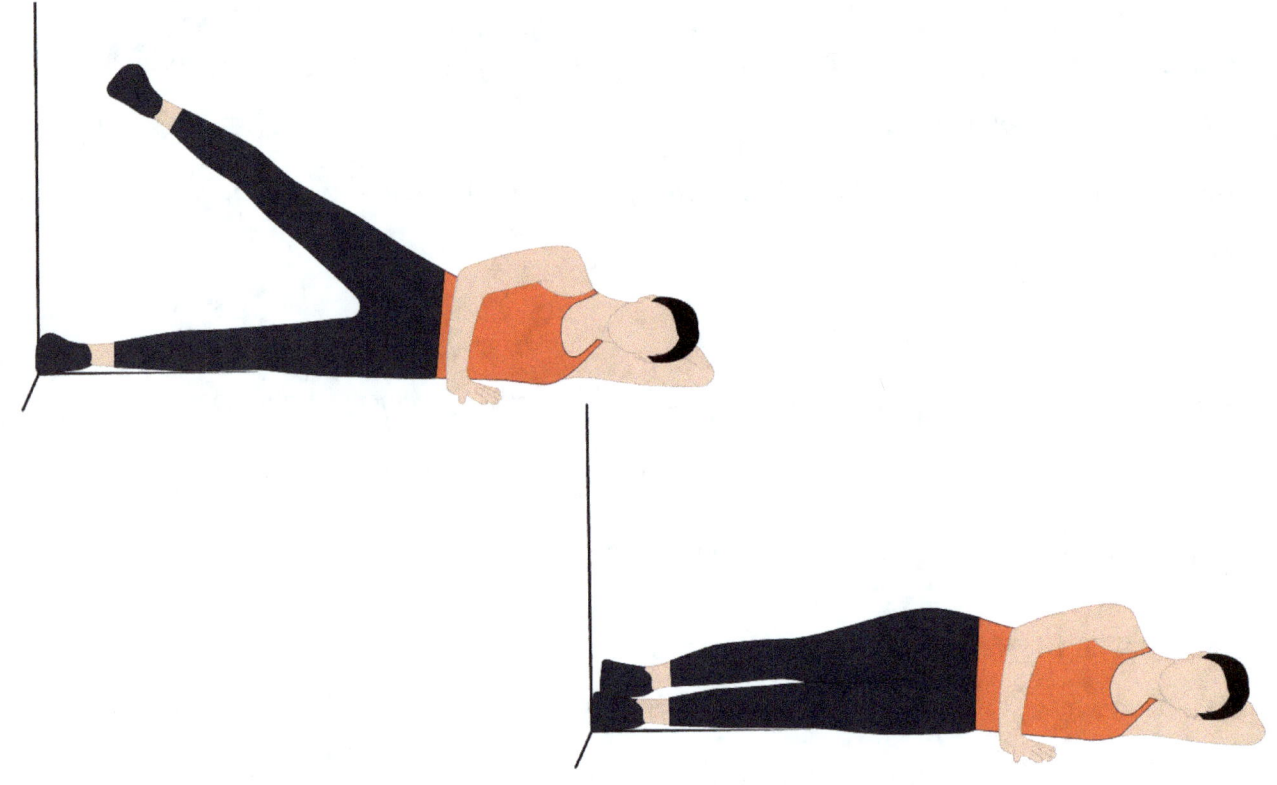

How to do Wall Side Leg Lifts:

1. Setup:

   o Lie on your side with your hips and back against a wall. Your legs should be extended straight out, parallel to the wall.

   o Ensure your head, shoulders, and hips are in alignment to maintain proper posture.

   o You can rest your bottom arm under your head for support and your top arm can be placed on your hip or stretched out for balance.

2. Positioning:

   o Stack your legs on top of each other.

   o Flex your feet, keeping them in line with your body.

3. Execution:

   o While keeping your back and hips against the wall, slowly lift your top leg upward as high as you comfortably can.

   o Ensure you are engaging your core muscles to maintain stability throughout the movement.

   o Hold the lifted position briefly, then slowly lower your leg back down to meet the bottom leg.

- o Repeat the lift for the desired number of repetitions, then switch sides.

4. Breathing:

- o Inhale as you lift your leg.
- o Exhale as you lower your leg back down.

5. Tips:

- o Focus on controlled movements rather than speed to maximize the effectiveness of the exercise.
- o Avoid arching your back or letting your hips roll forward or backward during the movement.
- o Keep your core engaged throughout to stabilize your body and protect your lower back.

- o If you find it challenging to keep your balance, you can place a hand on the floor in front of you for support.
- o Start with a small number of repetitions and gradually increase as you build strength and endurance.

6. Variations:

- o To increase intensity, you can add ankle weights or resistance bands around your thighs.
- o To target different muscles, you can experiment with slight variations in foot positioning or angle of the leg lift.
- o You can also perform this exercise in a standing position, leaning against the wall for support, if lying down is uncomfortable or not feasible.

Tips for Wall Side Leg Lifts:

- Focus on keeping the lifted leg straight and avoid bending at the knee during the movement.

- Keep your torso upright and avoid leaning or twisting excessively to ensure proper muscle engagement.

- Use the wall for balance but aim to rely on your leg muscles to lift and control the movement.

Benefits of Wall Side Leg Lifts:

- Targeted Muscle Engagement: Focuses on strengthening the outer thigh muscles (abductors), hips, and glutes.

- Enhanced Hip Stability: Improves hip stability and flexibility, which can be beneficial for various daily movements and activities.

- Low-Impact Exercise: Provides a low-impact option to strengthen and tone the outer thigh muscles without placing stress on the joints.

21. Wall Crunches

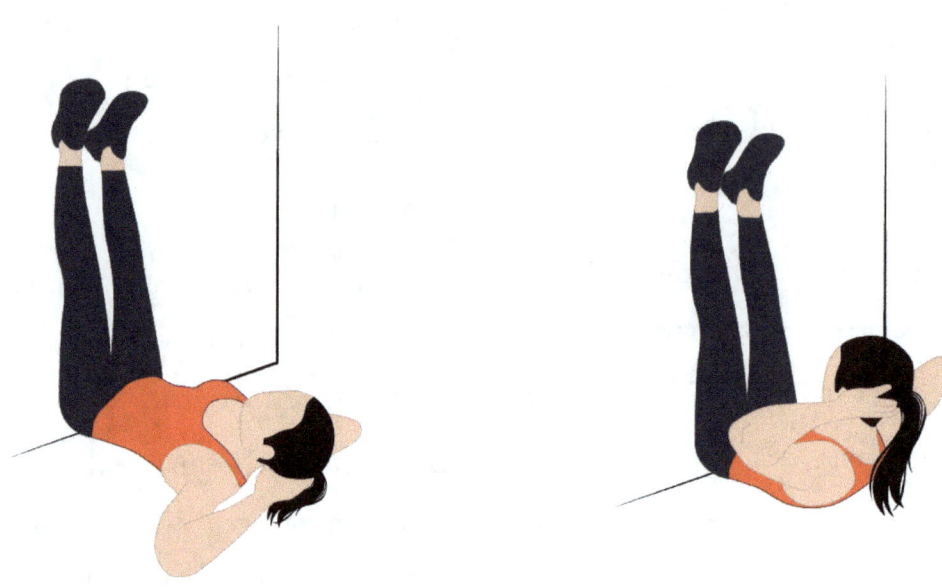

How to do Wall Crunches:

1. Starting Position: Lie on your back on the floor, and your legs flat against the wall.

2. Hand Positioning: Place your hands lightly behind your head, supporting your neck without pulling on it. Keep your elbows wide and avoid interlacing your fingers.

3. Engage Core Muscles: Engage your core by drawing your navel toward your spine. This helps maintain stability throughout the exercise.

4. Performing the Crunch:

    o Lift your head, neck, and shoulders slightly off the ground, gently pressing your lower back into the floor.

    o Contract your abdominal muscles, and imagine bringing your rib cage towards your pelvis as you lift your upper back off the ground.

5. Breathing and Pace: Exhale as you crunch upwards, inhale as you lower your upper back back down towards the floor. Keep a controlled pace throughout the movement.

6. Repetition: Continue performing the crunches for a set number of repetitions or a specific duration, focusing on quality and control of the movement.

Tips for Wall Crunches:

- Focus on using your abdominal muscles to lift your upper body rather than pulling on your neck with your hands.

- Keep your lower back pressed against the floor throughout the movement to engage the core effectively and prevent strain.

- Avoid using momentum; perform the exercise in a slow and controlled manner.

Benefits of Wall Crunches:

- Abdominal Strengthening: Targets the rectus abdominis muscles effectively.

- Improved Core Stability: Enhances core strength and stability, which is beneficial for posture and daily movements.

- Accessible Variation: Offers a modified version of crunches against a wall, which can be more comfortable for some individuals.

22. Wall Russian Twists

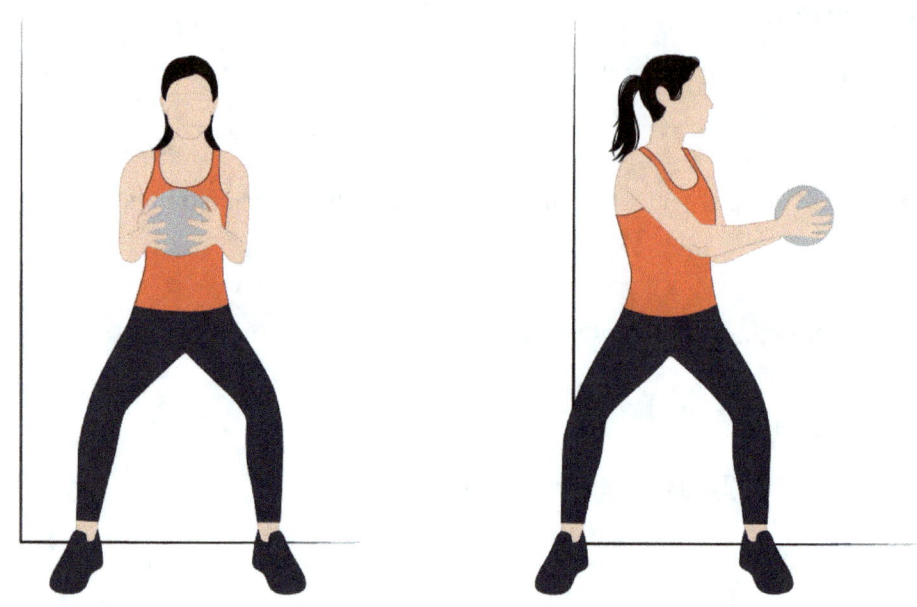

How to do Wall Russian Twists:

1. Find a Wall: Stand with your back against a sturdy wall, ensuring that you have enough space around you to rotate your torso freely.

2. Position Your Feet: Place your feet shoulder-width apart and a few inches away from the wall. Keep your knees slightly bent to maintain a stable stance.

3. Engage Your Core: Tighten your abdominal muscles to stabilize your torso and maintain proper posture throughout the exercise.

4. Extend Your Arms: Extend your arms straight out in front of you at shoulder height. Your palms should be facing each other, and your arms should be parallel to the ground.

5. Rotate Your Torso: Keeping your back against the wall, slowly rotate your torso to one side, bringing your arms and hands with you. Aim to rotate as far as comfortably possible without straining.

6. Twist to the Opposite Side: After reaching the end of your range of motion on one side, slowly rotate your torso back to the center. Then, rotate in the opposite direction, twisting your torso to the other side.

7. Focus on Control: Focus on controlling the movement with your core muscles rather than relying solely on momentum. Move slowly and deliberately to maximize the effectiveness of the exercise.

8. Maintain Proper Posture: Throughout the exercise, keep your back flat against the wall and avoid arching or rounding your spine. Your head should be in line with your spine, and your gaze should be forward.

9. Breathe: Coordinate your breathing with your movements. Exhale as you twist your torso to one side and inhale as you return to the center before twisting to the other side.

10. Repeat: Continue alternating twists from side to side for the desired number of repetitions or time duration. Aim for 10-15 repetitions per side to start, and adjust as needed based on your fitness level.

11. Cool Down: After completing the exercise, take a moment to relax and stretch your core muscles. You can perform gentle stretches such as a standing side stretch or a seated torso twist to release any tension.

Tips for Wall Russian Twists:

- Focus on engaging the core muscles to initiate and control the twisting motion.

- Keep your back straight and avoid slouching or rounding the spine during the exercise.

- Twist from your waist, not just your arms, to maximize the engagement of the obliques.

Benefits of Wall Russian Twists:

- Oblique Strengthening: Targets and strengthens the oblique muscles effectively.

- Improved Core Stability: Enhances core strength and stability, which is beneficial for posture and rotational movements.

- Accessible Variation: Offers a modified version of Russian twists against a wall, providing support for the lower back.

23. Wall Arm Circles

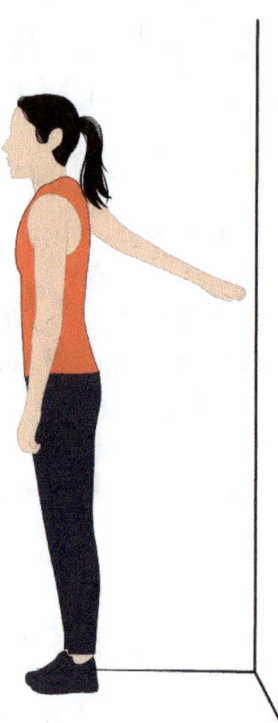

How to do Wall Arm Circles:

1. Setup:

   o Stand with your feet shoulder-width apart, facing the wall.

   o Position yourself so that one shoulder is touching the wall while the other shoulder is slightly away from the wall.

   o Keep your spine straight and engage your core muscles for stability.

2. Arm Positioning: extend your arm out to the sides, parallel to the floor.

3. Execution:

   o Begin by making small circular motions with your arms while keeping your shoulders pressed against the wall.

   o Gradually increase the size of the circles as you warm up and feel more comfortable with the movement.

   o Continue circling your arms for the desired number of repetitions or time.

4. Breathing:

   o Inhale as you bring your arms forward and upward.

   o Exhale as you circle your arms backward and downward.

5. Tips:

- Focus on maintaining contact between the shoulder touching the wall and the wall itself throughout the exercise.

- Keep your movements controlled and smooth, avoiding any jerky motions.

- Pay attention to any discomfort or strain in your shoulders, and adjust the size of your arm circles accordingly.

- If you have limited shoulder mobility, you can start with smaller circles and gradually work your way up to larger ones as your flexibility improves.

- Keep your neck relaxed and avoid shrugging your shoulders upward as you perform the circles.

- Perform the exercise at a pace that feels comfortable for you, and don't push yourself beyond your limits.

6. Variations:

- To target different muscles in the shoulders, you can vary the direction of the arm circles. For example, you can perform circles moving forward, backward, or in a combination of both.

- You can also increase the intensity of the exercise by holding light dumbbells in each hand while performing the arm circles.

- If standing is uncomfortable, you can perform this exercise in a seated position with your back against a wall for support.

Tips for Wall Arm Circles:

- Keep your movements controlled and deliberate, avoiding excessive swinging or jerking motions.

- Maintain proper posture throughout the exercise, keeping your core engaged and avoiding arching or rounding your back.

- Adjust the circle size according to your comfort level and gradually increase it as your shoulder mobility improves.

Benefits of Wall Arm Circles:

- Shoulder Warm-up: Helps warm up and increase blood flow to the shoulder muscles before workouts or activities.

- Improved Shoulder Mobility: Enhances shoulder joint mobility and flexibility.

- Muscle Activation: Engages the muscles of the shoulders, arms, and upper back.

24. Wall Angel

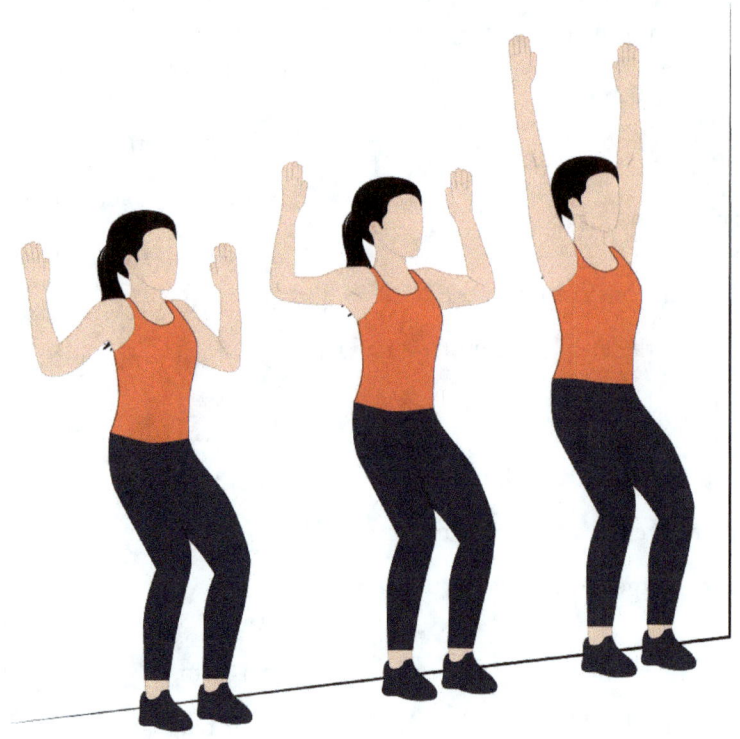

How to do Wall Angels:

1. Starting Position: Stand with your back against a flat wall, making sure your feet are a few inches away from the wall. Ensure your head, upper back, and hips are touching the wall.

2. Hand Positioning: Bend your elbows at a 90-degree angle, so your upper arms are parallel to the ground, and your forearms point upward. Your hands and elbows should also be touching the wall.

3. Engage Core Muscles: Engage your core by drawing your navel toward your spine. This helps maintain stability throughout the exercise.

4. Performing the Movement:

    o Slowly slide your arms upward along the wall, keeping your elbows and hands in contact with the wall at all times.

    o Extend your arms as high as you comfortably can overhead while maintaining contact with the wall.

    o Keep your shoulder blades pinned against the wall and try to press your lower back into the wall throughout the movement.

- Return your arms to the starting position, sliding them back down the wall while maintaining contact with your elbows, forearms, and hands.

5. Repeat the Motion: Perform this sliding movement up and down the wall, creating a motion that resembles making "snow angels" on the wall.

6. Breathing: Exhale as you slide your arms up, inhale as you bring them back down.

Tips for Wall Angels:

- Focus on maintaining contact between your head, upper back, elbows, forearms, and hands with the wall throughout the movement.

- Move slowly and with control, emphasizing the range of motion that feels comfortable and avoiding any discomfort or strain.

- Engage your core muscles to stabilize your body against the wall.

Benefits of Wall Angels:

- Posture Improvement: Helps improve posture by promoting proper alignment of the shoulders and upper back.

- Shoulder Mobility: Enhances shoulder mobility and flexibility by stretching and strengthening the muscles around the shoulder blades.

- Upper Back Strengthening: Engages the muscles of the upper back, contributing to improved upper body strength and stability.

25. Standing Glute Kickbacks

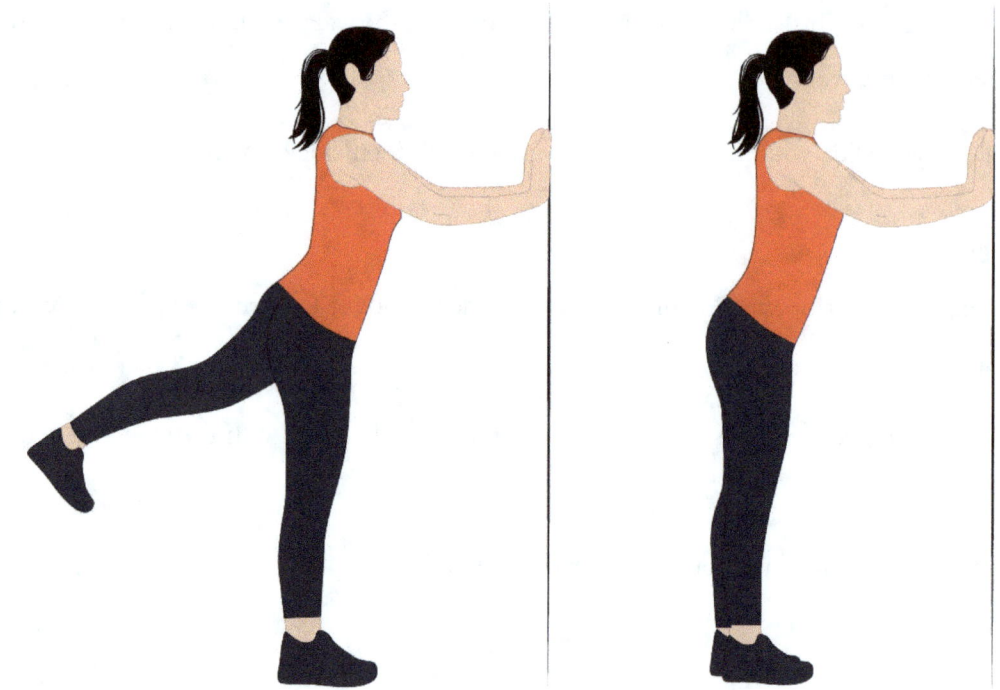

How to do Standing Glute Kickbacks:

1. Starting Position: Stand upright with your feet shoulder-width apart. Engage your core by drawing your navel toward your spine for stability.

2. Hand Positioning: Place your hands on the wall for support.

3. Performing the Kickback:

    o   Shift your weight onto one leg and slightly bend the knee.

    o   Lift the opposite leg behind you, keeping the knee straight, while maintaining a neutral spine.

    o   Focus on using your glute muscles to lift the leg as high as comfortable without arching your back or leaning excessively forward.

4. Squeeze and Lower: At the top of the movement, pause briefly and squeeze your glutes to activate them.

5. Return to Starting Position: Lower your leg back down with control to the starting position, maintaining control throughout the movement.

6. Repetition: Perform the desired number of repetitions on one leg before switching to the other side.

Tips for Standing Glute Kickbacks:

- Maintain a stable and controlled movement throughout without swinging the leg or using momentum.

- Keep your hips squared and avoid rotating them as you lift your leg.

- Focus on the contraction of the glute muscles at the top of the movement.

Benefits of Standing Glute Kickbacks:

- Gluteal Strengthening: Targets and strengthens the glute muscles, particularly the gluteus maximus.

- Improved Hip Stability: Enhances hip stability and balance.

- Accessible Exercise: Requires minimal space and no equipment, making it easy to perform anywhere.

26. Wall Figure 4 Stretch

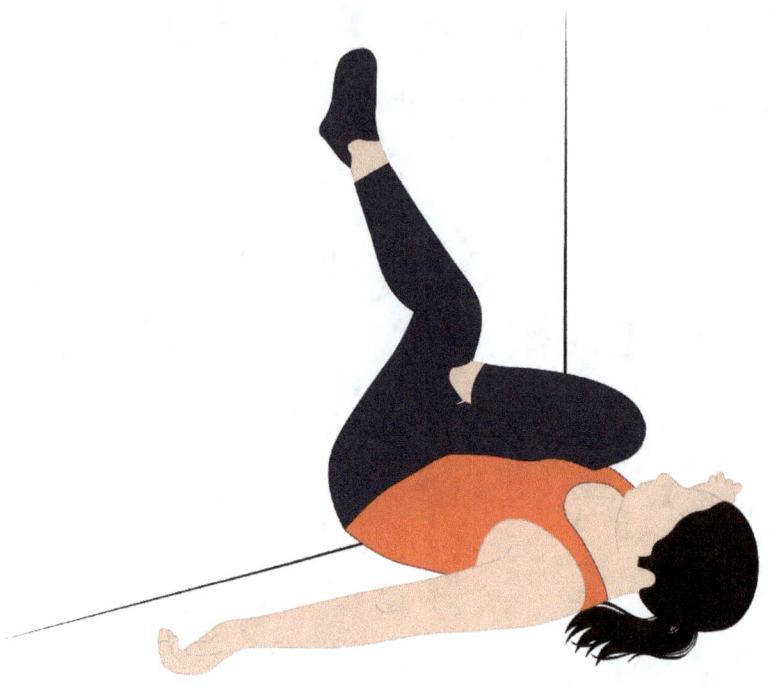

How to do Wall Figure 4 Stretch:

1. Starting Position: Lie on your back on the floor near a wall, with your knees bent and your feet flat on the ground.

2. Positioning the Legs:

    o Lift your right leg and place your right ankle on top of your left thigh, just above the knee, forming a "figure 4" shape with your legs.

    o Flex your right foot to protect your knee and gently push your right knee away from your body to open the hip.

3. Approaching the Wall:

    o Scoot closer to the wall while maintaining the figure 4 position with your legs.

    o Once close to the wall, lift your left foot and place it against the wall, bending your left knee to bring your shin parallel to the wall.

4. Adjustment for Comfort: You can modify the distance from the wall based on your comfort level. The closer your hips are to the wall, the deeper the stretch may feel.

5. Maintaining the Stretch:

- Relax into the stretch, allowing gravity and the wall to gently increase the sensation in the outer right hip and glute area.
- Breathe deeply and try to relax into the stretch for about 30 seconds to 1 minute.

6. Switching Sides: Release the stretch by uncrossing your legs, then repeat the same process on the other side by placing the left ankle on the right thigh and adjusting your position near the wall.

Tips for Wall Figure 4 Stretch:

- Pay attention to your comfort and avoid forcing the stretch beyond your limit. It should be a gentle, comfortable stretch, not a painful one.

- Keep your upper body relaxed and try to maintain a neutral spine during the stretch.

- Engage in deep, relaxed breathing to encourage relaxation and deepen the stretch.

Benefits of Wall Figure 4 Stretch:

- Glute and Hip Flexibility: Stretches the glute muscles and hip rotators, promoting flexibility and reducing tightness.

- Lower Back Relief: Helps alleviate tension in the lower back by targeting the hip and glute area.

- Improved Posture: Regular practice can contribute to better hip mobility and posture.

27. Standing Leg Circles

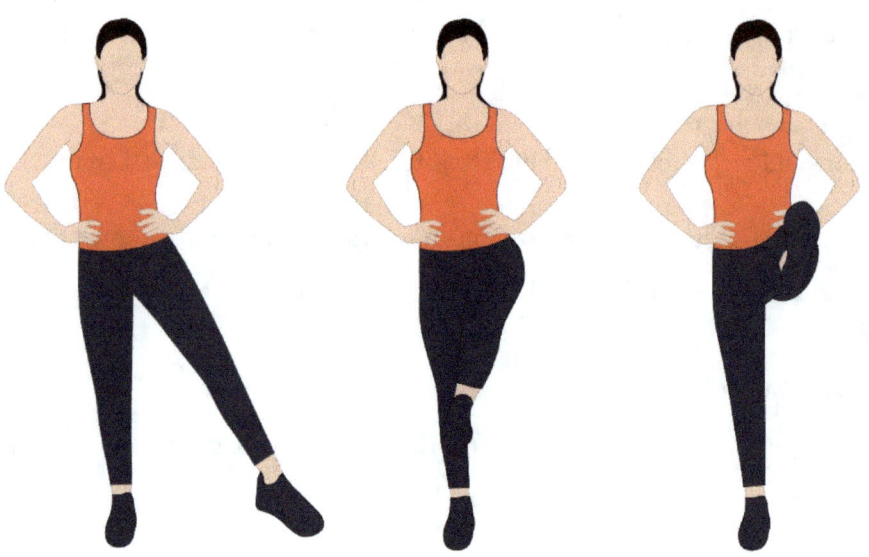

How to do Standing Leg Circles:

1. Starting Position: Stand tall with your feet together and engage your core by drawing your navel toward your spine for stability.

2. Hand Positioning: Place your hands on your hips or hold onto a stable surface, like a chair or countertop, for balance if needed.

3. Performing the Leg Circles:

    o Lift one leg off the ground, keeping it straight and slightly to the side of your body.

    o Begin to make circular motions with your lifted leg, moving from the hip joint. Perform clockwise or counterclockwise circles, depending on your preference.

    o Maintain control and aim for a full range of motion without rotating your torso excessively or leaning to one side.

4. Controlled Movement:

- Focus on the movement coming from your hip joint rather than your entire leg. Keep your hips and upper body stable.

- Ensure that your supporting leg remains straight but with a slight bend in the knee for balance.

5. Repetition: Complete a set number of circles in one direction with one leg before switching to the other leg and performing circles in the opposite direction.

6. Switching Legs: Once finished with one leg, switch to the other leg and perform leg circles in both directions.

Tips for Standing Leg Circles:

- Maintain a stable and controlled movement without swinging your leg or using momentum.

- Keep your torso upright and avoid leaning or twisting excessively.

- Start with small circles and gradually increase the size of the circles as your range of motion improves.

Benefits of Standing Leg Circles:

- Hip Mobility: Improves hip joint mobility by engaging and strengthening the hip muscles.

- Muscle Activation: Targets the hip abductors, flexors, and stabilizing muscles of the leg.

- Balance and Stability: Enhances balance and stability by engaging the core and supporting leg.

28. Wall Dead Bug

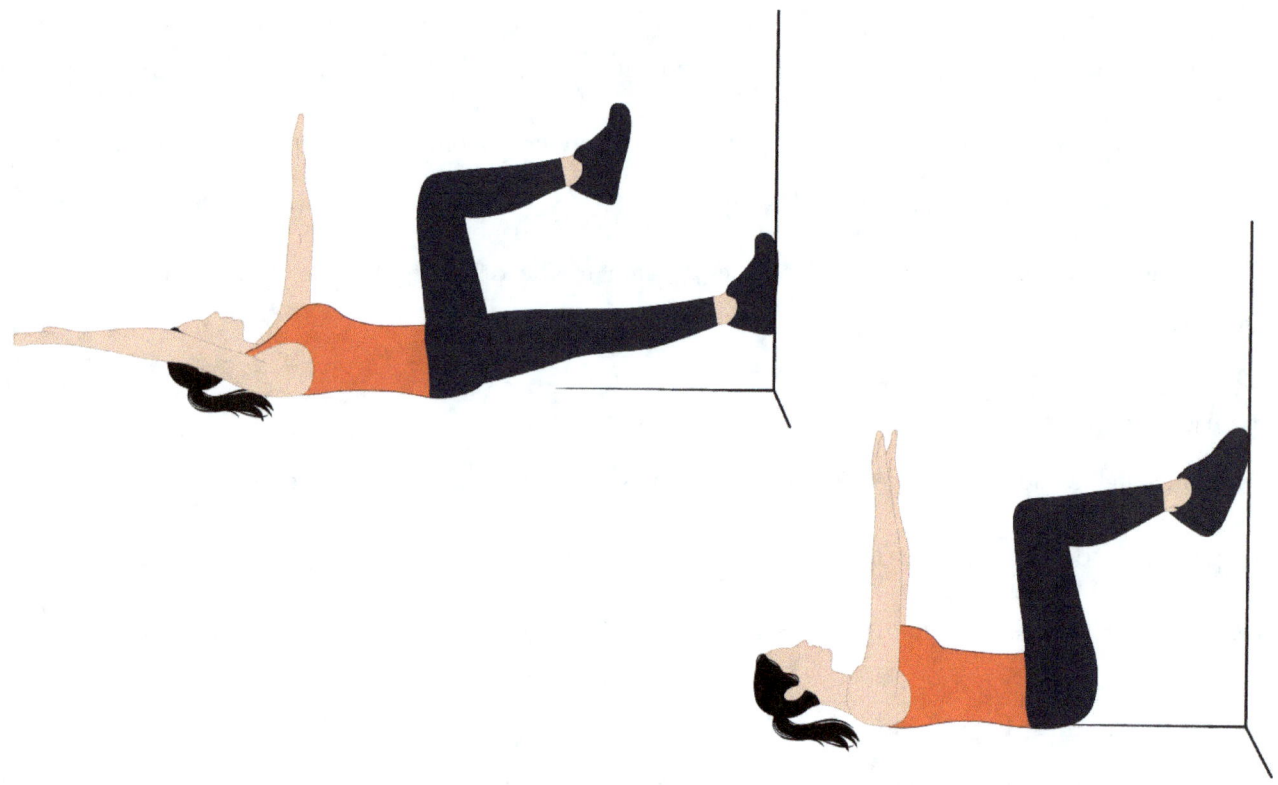

How to do Wall Dead Bug:

1. Starting Position: Lie on your back on the floor with your feet against a wall and your knees bent at a 90-degree angle, so your shins are parallel to the ground.

2. Engage Core Muscles: Engage your core by drawing your navel toward your spine. This helps maintain stability throughout the exercise.

3. Arm Positioning: Extend your arms straight up towards the ceiling, palms facing each other.

4. Performing the Exercise:

   o Simultaneously lower your right arm towards the floor, while straightening your left leg and lowering it towards the ground, keeping it in contact with the wall.

   o Pause briefly when your arm and leg are close to the ground but do not let them touch.

   o Return your arm and leg to the starting position simultaneously, bringing your right arm back up and bending your left knee, bringing it back to the starting position.

5. Switching Sides:

- Alternate the movement, lowering your left arm and right leg while keeping the opposite arm and leg stable against the wall.
- Repeat the exercise, alternating sides for the desired number of repetitions.

6. Breathing: Exhale as you extend your arm and leg, inhale as you return to the starting position.

Tips for Wall Dead Bug:

- Maintain contact between the arm and leg with the wall throughout the movement.

- Keep your lower back pressed against the floor to engage the core effectively and prevent strain.

- Perform the exercise slowly and with control to maximize engagement and stability.

Benefits of Wall Dead Bug:

- Core Strengthening: Targets the deep core muscles, including the rectus abdominis and transversus abdominis.

- Improved Stability: Enhances core stability and coordination between the upper and lower body.

- Low Back Support: Can help in developing strength and stability in the lower back muscles.

29. Wall Hip Flexor Stretches

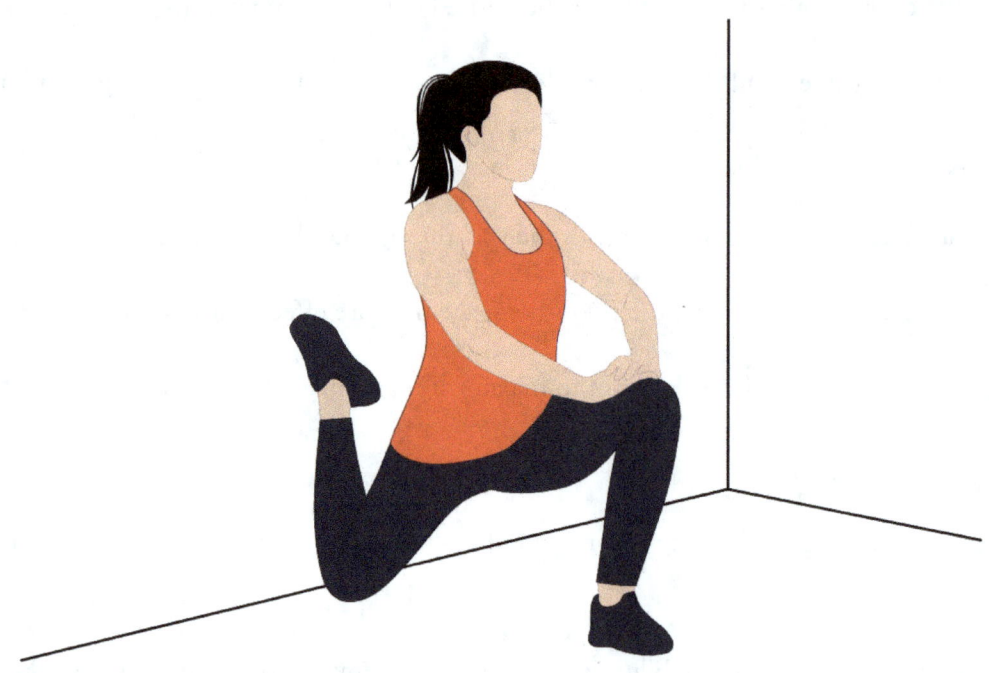

How to do Wall Hip Flexor Stretch:

1. Starting Position: Begin in a half-kneeling position facing away from a wall. Place a cushion or mat on the ground for knee comfort. Your front knee should be at a 90-degree angle, aligned with your ankle, and your back knee should also be bent at a 90-degree angle with your toes tucked under for support.

2. Positioning Against the Wall: Gently lean back and place the top of your back foot against the wall behind you. Your shin and the top of your foot should be flat against the wall, creating a stable base.

3. Engage Core Muscles: Engage your core by drawing your navel toward your spine. This helps maintain stability throughout the stretch.

4. Performing the Stretch:

    o Keeping your torso upright and without arching your back, gently shift your hips forward to feel a stretch in the front of your back hip (the hip flexor of the leg that's back).

    o Ensure you're not overarching your lower back or leaning excessively forward.

5. Hold and Breathe: Hold the stretch for about 20 to 30 seconds while breathing deeply and relaxing into the stretch. Avoid holding your breath.

6. Switching Sides: Release the stretch and switch to stretch the other side by switching your leg positions and repeating the same steps.

Tips for Wall Hip Flexor Stretch:

- Focus on feeling a comfortable stretch in the front of the hip without any sharp or painful sensations.

- Keep your movements controlled and avoid leaning too far forward or excessively arching your lower back.

- Increase the stretch gradually if it feels comfortable, but do not force the movement beyond your comfort level.

Benefits of Wall Hip Flexor Stretch:

- Hip Flexor Release: Helps to lengthen and release tension in the hip flexor muscles.

- Improved Hip Mobility: Enhances flexibility and range of motion in the hip area.

- Posture Improvement: Can contribute to better posture by addressing tightness in the hip flexors caused by prolonged sitting.

30. Standing Wall Twist

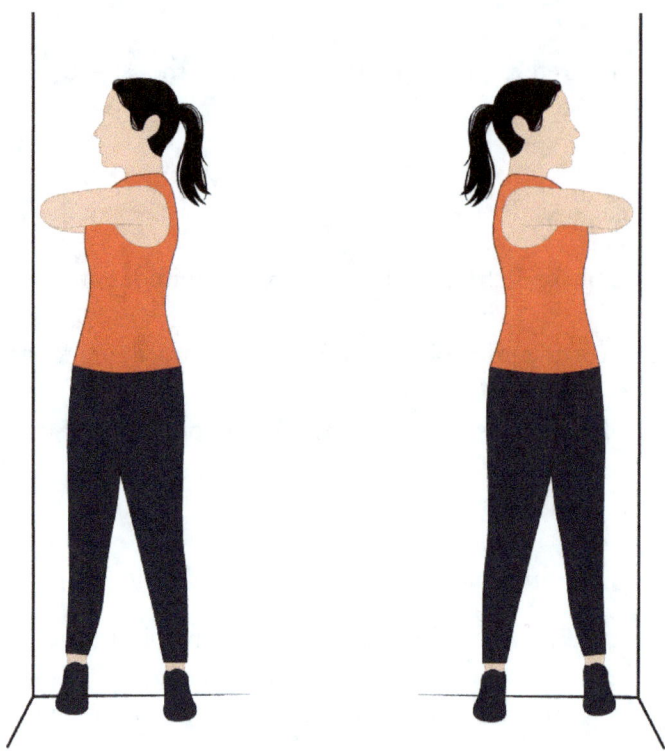

How to do Standing Wall Twist:

1. Starting Position: Stand tall with your feet about hip-width apart, facing away from the wall. Keep your spine straight and your shoulders relaxed.

2. Arm Positioning: make your elbows bent 90-degree.

3. Performing the Twist:

    o Without moving your feet, begin to rotate your upper body to the right, twisting from your torso while keeping your hips facing forward.

    o As you twist, follow your right hand with your gaze, looking over your right shoulder.

4. Maintain the Twist: Hold the twist position for a few seconds, feeling the stretch through your torso and spine.

5. Return to Center: Slowly unwind from the twist, bringing your torso back to the center-facing position.

6. Switching Sides: Repeat the twist in the opposite direction, rotating your upper body to the left while keeping your hips stationary.

7. Breathing: Inhale as you return to the center, exhale as you twist to each side.

8. Repetition: Repeat the twisting motion, alternating from side to side for several repetitions or as desired.

Tips for Standing Wall Twist:

- Keep your hips and lower body stable without allowing them to rotate; the twist should come from your upper torso.

- Perform the movement in a slow, controlled manner to avoid any sudden jerks or strains.

- Focus on maintaining good posture throughout the exercise, keeping your spine elongated.

Benefits of Standing Wall Twist:

- Spinal Mobility: Improves flexibility and mobility of the spine, particularly in the thoracic region.

- Core Engagement: Engages the core muscles, including the obliques, to support and stabilize the twisting motion.

- Postural Awareness: Helps in enhancing awareness of posture and encourages a full range of motion in the upper body.

31 Wall Side Lunges

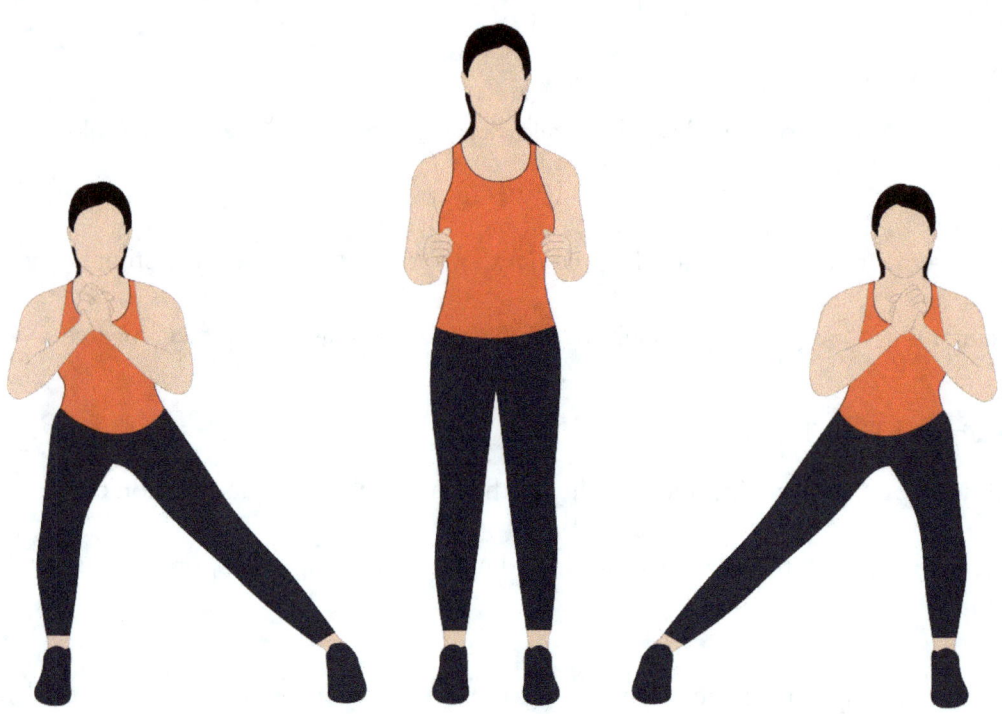

How to do Wall Side Lunges:

1. Starting Position: Stand upright with your side facing a wall, about an arm's length away. Keep your feet wider than shoulder-width apart, toes pointed forward.

2. Hand Positioning: Place your hands on your hips for balance or extend them in front of you for added stability.

3. Performing the Lunge:

   o Shift your body weight to one side, bending that knee while keeping the other leg straight.

   o Lower your body by pushing your hips back and bending the knee of the side you shifted your weight towards, as if you're sitting back into a chair. Keep your back straight and your chest lifted.

4. Maintain Stability: The foot of your bent leg should remain flat on the floor while the other leg stays straight with the foot planted firmly on the ground.

5. Depth of the Lunge: Lower your body until your thigh is close to parallel with the floor, if possible, while ensuring your knee does not extend past your toes.

6. Return to Starting Position: Push through the heel of the bent leg to return to the starting position, engaging the inner thigh and glute muscles.

7. Switch Sides: Repeat the same movement on the other side, alternating between left and right sides.

8. Repetition: Perform the desired number of repetitions for each side, focusing on controlled movements and proper form.

Tips for Wall Side Lunges:

- Keep your back straight and your chest lifted throughout the movement to maintain good posture.

- Ensure proper alignment by tracking your knee over your toes without allowing it to extend past the toes.

- Engage your core muscles for stability and balance during the lunges.

Benefits of Wall Side Lunges:

- Targets Inner and Outer Thighs: Engages and strengthens the adductor and abductor muscles of the thighs.

- Glute Activation: Works the glute muscles while performing the side lunging motion.

- Improves Hip Mobility: Helps in enhancing hip flexibility and mobility.

32. Wall Walks

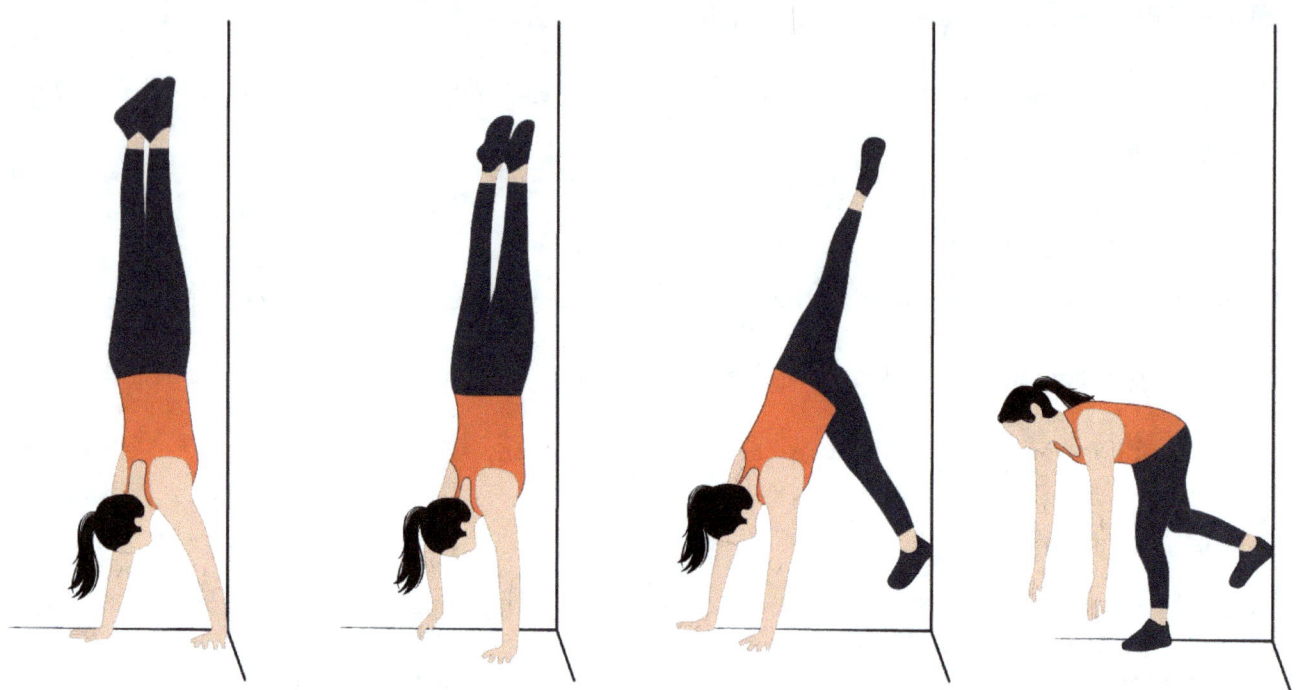

How to do Wall Walks:

1. Starting Position: Begin in a high plank position facing away from the wall, with your feet against the wall and your hands shoulder-width apart on the floor.

2. Walk Your Feet Up the Wall: Slowly start walking your feet up the wall while simultaneously walking your hands backward towards the wall. Keep your core engaged and maintain a straight body line.

3. Walk Until in a Vertical Position: Continue walking your feet up the wall and your hands towards the wall until your body is in an inverted position with your arms fully extended, resembling an upward-facing position.

4. Hold the Inverted Position: Once in a vertical position, hold it a few seconds, engaging your core, shoulders, and arms to stabilize your body.

5. Walk Back Down: Carefully reverse the movement by walking your hands forward away from the wall and walking your feet down the wall until you return to the starting plank position.

6. Repetition: Repeat the wall walk movement for the desired number of reps or for a specific duration.

Tips for Wall Walks:

- Maintain a tight core throughout the exercise to prevent your lower back from arching excessively.

- Engage your shoulders and arms to support your body weight while transitioning into the inverted position.

- Focus on controlled movements and avoid rushing through the exercise.

Benefits of Wall Walks:

- Full-Body Workout: Engages the upper body, core, shoulders, and stabilizing muscles, offering a comprehensive workout.

- Shoulder and Core Strength: Builds strength in the shoulders, arms, and core muscles.

- Improves Stability: Enhances overall stability and balance.

33. Wall Sprints (high knees against the wall)

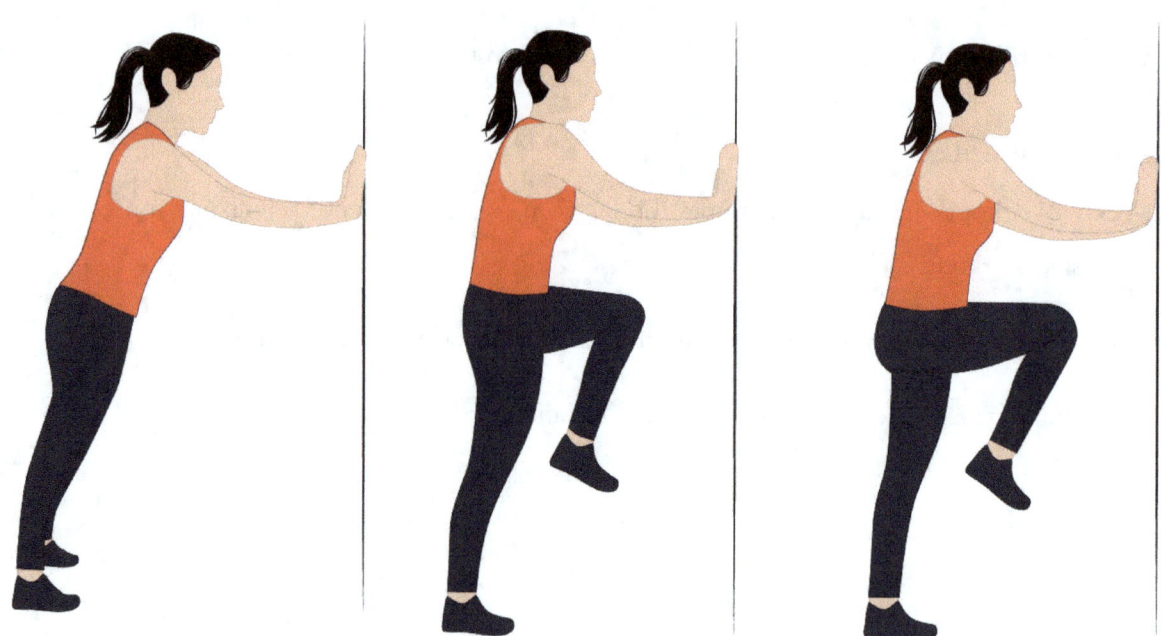

How to do Wall Sprints (High Knees Against the Wall):

1. Starting Position: Stand facing a wall with your feet hip-width apart and arms by your sides.

2. Positioning Against the Wall: Lean forward slightly and place your hands flat against the wall at shoulder height, slightly wider than shoulder-width apart. Your arms should be fully extended.

3. Engage Core Muscles: Engage your core by drawing your navel toward your spine for stability throughout the exercise.

4. Performing the Exercise:

    o   Start running in place, lifting your knees as high as possible towards your chest alternately.

    o   Drive one knee up towards your chest while the other leg extends behind you, pushing off the ground as if sprinting.

    o   Maintain a rapid but controlled pace, continuously switching legs as you "sprint" against the wall.

5. Arms Movement: Keep your arms pumping back and forth in sync with your legs, mimicking a natural running motion.

6. Repetition: Continue the high-knee sprinting motion against the wall for the desired duration or a specific number of repetitions.

Tips for Wall Sprints:

- Ensure your hands remain in contact with the wall throughout the exercise to provide support and stability.

- Focus on lifting your knees as high as possible while maintaining a quick pace.

- Keep your upper body upright and avoid leaning too far forward or backward.

Benefits of Wall Sprints:

- Cardiovascular Workout: Provides a cardiovascular challenge similar to sprinting, improving heart rate and endurance.

- Lower Body Strength: Engages and strengthens the lower body muscles, including the quadriceps, hamstrings, and hip flexors.

- Core Engagement: Involves the core muscles to stabilize the body during the high-knee motion.

34. Wall Splits

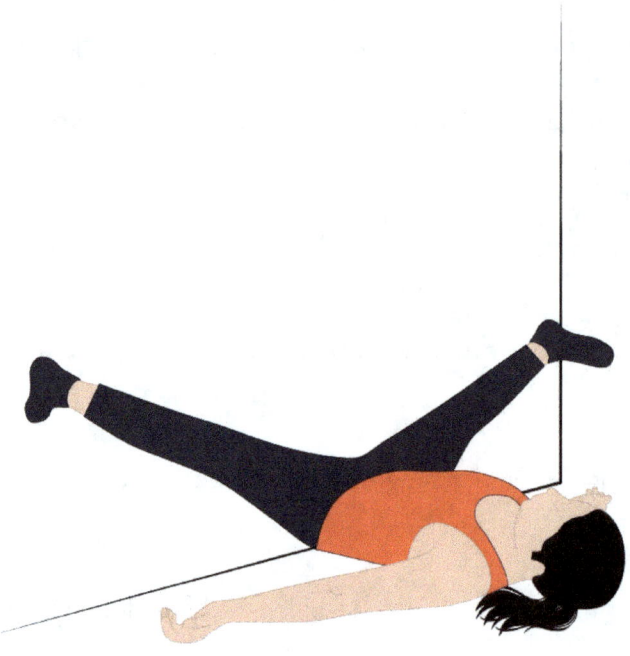

How to do Wall Splits:

1. Find a Wall:

    - Locate a clear wall space where you have enough room to perform the split comfortably and safely.

    - Place a yoga mat or cushion on the floor for added comfort.

2. Starting Position:

    - Sit on the floor with your side facing the wall.

    - Lie down on your back and swing your legs up against the wall, ensuring your buttocks are as close to the wall as possible. Your legs should be straight and pressed against the wall.

3. Opening Your Legs: slowly begin to open your legs into a straddle position by sliding them down the wall. Keep your feet flexed to protect your knees and engage your core for stability.

4. Finding Your Limit: move your legs down the wall gradually, only as far as your flexibility allows. Stop at a point where you feel a deep stretch but no pain or discomfort.

5. Hold the Position: once you've reached a comfortable stretch, hold the wall split position for about 30 seconds to 1 minute while breathing deeply and relaxing into the stretch.

6. Gradual Progression: over time, aim to increase the depth of your split gradually, moving your legs further down the wall as your flexibility improves.

Tips for Wall Splits:

- Perform this stretch after a proper warm-up to ensure your muscles are adequately prepared for deep stretching.

- Focus on relaxing your muscles and breathing deeply to ease into the stretch gradually.

- Never force yourself into a split position beyond your comfort level to avoid injury.

Benefits of Wall Splits:

- Improved Flexibility: Helps in stretching the hamstrings, groin, hips, and inner thighs to enhance overall flexibility.

- Muscle Relaxation: Allows for the release of tension in the lower body muscles, promoting relaxation.

- Increased Range of Motion: Regular practice can lead to increased range of motion in the legs and hips.

35. Wall Tricep Stretch

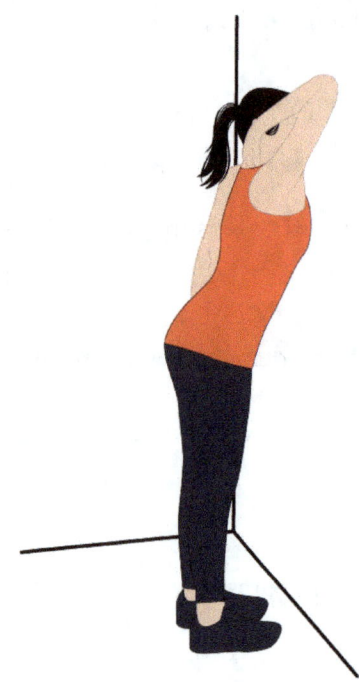

How to do Wall Tricep Stretch:

1. Starting Position:

    o Stand facing a wall or another sturdy vertical surface.

    o Raise your right arm straight up, reaching towards the ceiling.

2. Positioning the Arm:

    o Bend your right elbow and place your right hand behind your upper back, between your shoulder blades, with your palm facing your upper back.

    o Try to slide your right hand as far down your back as comfortably possible.

3. Using the Wall:

    o Lean your body slightly against the wall with your right elbow pointing towards the ceiling.

    o Rest your right elbow against the wall at about shoulder height.

4. Stretching the Tricep:

- Gently push your right forearm and hand down the center of your upper back, feeling a stretch in the back of your right arm (tricep muscle).
- Avoid arching your back excessively during the stretch; try to keep your spine in a neutral position.

5. Hold and Breathe:

- Hold the stretch for about 20-30 seconds, while breathing deeply and relaxing into the stretch.
- Avoid any sharp pain; it should be a gentle, comfortable stretch.

6. Switching Sides: release the stretch and switch to stretch the left tricep by repeating the same steps with your left arm.

Tips for Wall Tricep Stretch:

- Ensure your movements are controlled and avoid any sudden or jerky motions to prevent injury.

- If you can't reach your hand to your upper back, you can use a towel or a strap to bridge the gap between your hands and gently pull on the towel for a stretch.

Benefits of Wall Tricep Stretch:

- Tricep Flexibility: Improves flexibility in the triceps muscle, which can help with various upper body movements.

- Posture Improvement: Stretching the triceps can contribute to better posture and shoulder mobility.

- Reduces Muscle Tension: Relaxes and reduces tension in the triceps, especially after workouts involving the arms.

36. Wall Squats level 2

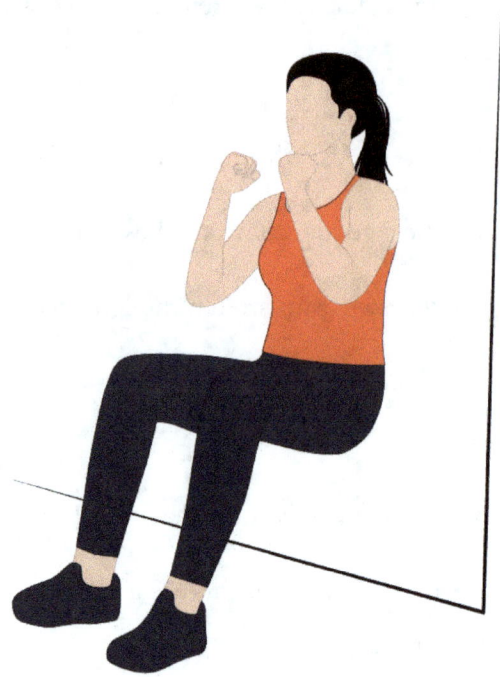

How to do Wall Squats (Wall Sits):

1. Starting Position:

    o Stand with your back against a wall and your feet positioned slightly wider than shoulder-width apart.

    o Your feet should be about 1-2 feet away from the wall.

2. Lowering into the Squat:

    o Slowly slide your back down the wall, bending your knees until your thighs are parallel to the floor.

    o Keep your back straight against the wall and ensure your knees are positioned directly above your ankles (not extending past your toes).

3. Form and Alignment:

    o Maintain a neutral spine with your shoulders relaxed against the wall.

    o Engage your core muscles to support your lower back throughout the exercise.

4. Hold the Squat Position: hold this seated position (squat) for as long as comfortable. Aim to hold it for at least 30 seconds to 1 minute, gradually increasing the duration over time.

5. Breathing: breathe deeply and evenly while holding the squat position to maintain relaxation and focus.

6. Returning to Starting Position: to come out of the squat, slowly push yourself up using your legs, straightening your knees and returning to a standing position.

Tips for Wall Squats:

- Focus on keeping your weight on your heels and avoid lifting your toes during the squat to engage the leg muscles effectively.

- Ensure your knees stay aligned with your toes and don't cave inward or extend past your toes to prevent unnecessary strain.

- Gradually increase the duration of the wall sit as your leg strength improves.

Benefits of Wall Squats:

- Leg Strength: Strengthens the quadriceps, hamstrings, glutes, and calf muscles.

- Endurance Building: Helps improve lower body endurance and stamina.

- Accessible Exercise: Requires minimal space and no equipment, making it easy to perform anywhere.

37. Wall Lateral Leg Swings

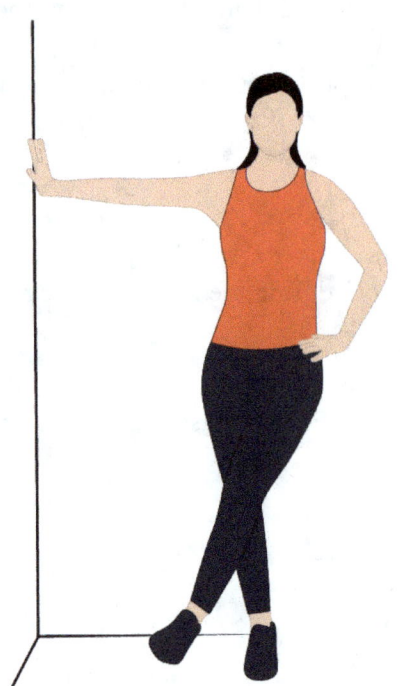 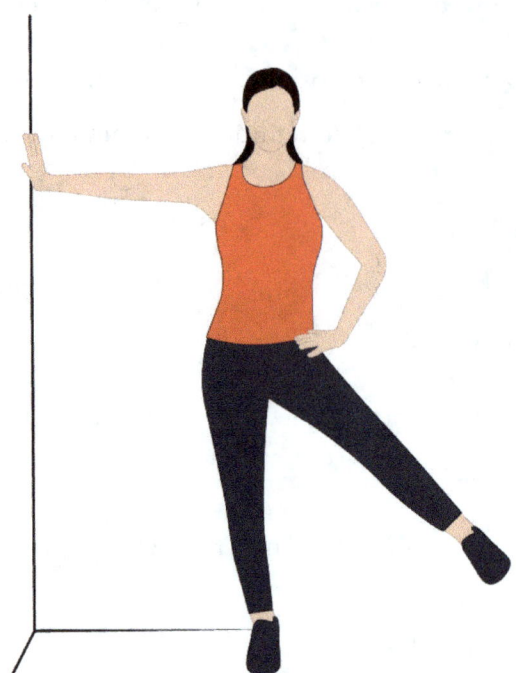

How to do Wall Lateral Leg Swings:

1. Starting Position:

    - Stand sideways to a wall, with one hand resting lightly on the wall for balance.

    - Stand tall with your feet together and your core engaged for stability.

2. Swinging Leg Outward:

    - Swing your outside leg (farthest from the wall) out to the side, keeping it straight and leading with your heel.

    - Swing your leg out as far as comfortable without leaning your upper body or compromising your balance.

3. Swinging Leg Inward:

    - After swinging your leg outward, bring it back across your body in a controlled motion, crossing in front of your standing leg.

    - Swing your leg inward toward the midline of your body, leading with the inner edge of your foot.

4. Repeat the Swings: perform the swinging motion back and forth, allowing your leg to move freely while maintaining control and stability through your core.

5. Switching Sides: after completing the desired number of swings on one side, turn around to face the other direction and repeat the exercise with the other leg.

6. Controlled Movement: Keep the swinging motion controlled and smooth, avoiding any jerky movements that could compromise balance.

Tips for Wall Lateral Leg Swings:

- Start with smaller swings and gradually increase the range of motion as your muscles warm up.

- Keep your standing leg slightly bent for better stability and engage your core to help maintain balance.

- Focus on controlling the movement and avoid using momentum to swing the leg.

Benefits of Wall Lateral Leg Swings:

- Hip Mobility: Helps improve hip flexibility and mobility, particularly in the hip abductors and adductors.

- Dynamic Stretching: Acts as a dynamic stretch for the legs, enhancing range of motion.

- Balance and Stability: Engages core muscles and promotes balance while strengthening the supporting leg.

38. Wall Side Stretch

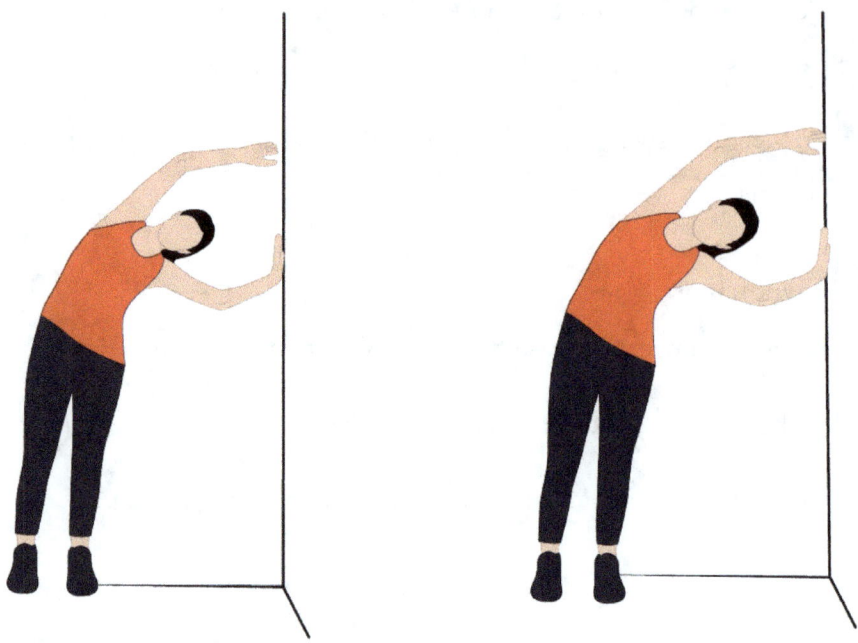

How to do Wall Side Stretch:

1. Starting Position:

   o   Stand tall next to a wall with your feet hip-width apart.

   o   Extend one arm up and reach towards the ceiling while keeping your feet planted firmly on the ground.

2. Hand Placement on the Wall: extend your arms and place your palms against the wall at shoulder height, with your fingertips pointing upward.

3. Performing the Stretch:

   o   Lean your body away from the wall towards the opposite side without bending forward or backward.

   o   Keep your arm straight and your shoulder pressed gently against the wall to feel a deep stretch along the side of your body.

4. Engage Core and Maintain Alignment:

   o   Engage your core muscles to prevent leaning excessively and to maintain a neutral spine.

- o Avoid arching your back or leaning forward during the stretch.

5. Feeling the Stretch:

- o You should feel a stretch along the entire side of your body, from your fingertips down to your hip.
- o Hold the stretch for about 20-30 seconds while breathing deeply and relaxing into the stretch.

6. Switching Sides: release the stretch and switch to stretch the opposite side by repeating the same steps with your other arm.

Tips for Wall Side Stretch:

- Focus on lengthening the entire side of your body while keeping your spine in a neutral position.

- Avoid any jerky or forceful movements; perform the stretch smoothly and gradually.

- Breathe deeply and consistently throughout the stretch to relax and allow for a deeper stretch.

Benefits of Wall Side Stretch:

- Oblique Stretch: Targets the oblique muscles, aiding in improving flexibility and reducing tension.

- Improved Range of Motion: Helps enhance the flexibility of the side body, including the intercostal muscles.

- Posture Support: Regular stretching of the side body muscles can contribute to better posture and reduce stiffness.

39. Wall Marches

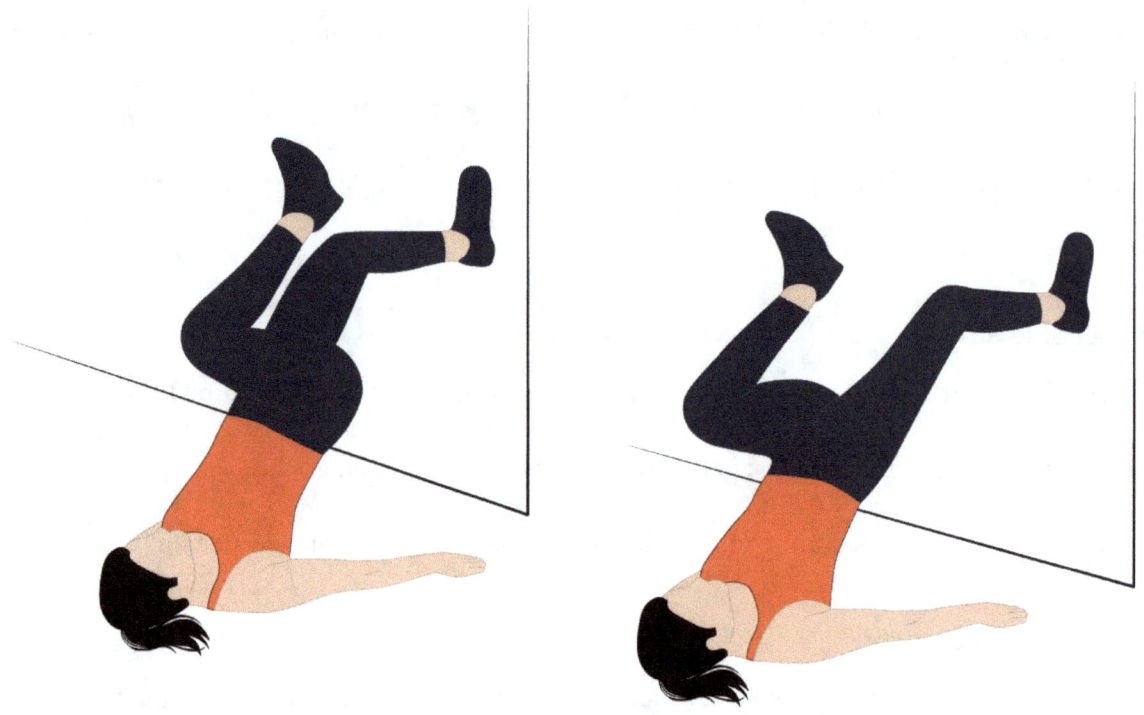

How to do Wall Marches:

1. Setup:

   o Lie on your back with your buttocks close to a wall. Your legs should be extended straight up against the wall, creating a 90-degree angle with your body.

   o Place your arms flat on the floor by your sides, palms down, for stability.

   o Engage your core muscles by pulling your belly button towards your spine.

2. Bridge Position:

   o Press your palms into the floor and lift your hips upward, creating a bridge position with your body. Your shoulders, hips, and knees should form a straight line.

   o Keep your neck relaxed and gaze towards the ceiling to maintain proper alignment.

3. Marching Movement:

   o From the bridge position, slowly lower one foot down the wall towards the floor while keeping the other leg in place.

- As you lower your leg, maintain the bridge position and avoid arching your back excessively.
- Once your foot reaches a few inches above the floor, reverse the movement and bring that foot back up the wall.
- As you return the first foot, begin lowering the opposite foot down the wall.
- Continue alternating legs in a marching motion, keeping the movement controlled and steady.

4. Breathing:
   - Inhale as you lower your foot down the wall.
   - Exhale as you lift your foot back up the wall.

5. Tips:
   - Focus on stability and control throughout the exercise, especially in the bridge position.
   - Keep your hips lifted and avoid sagging or dropping them towards the floor.
   - Maintain a neutral spine by engaging your core muscles and avoiding excessive arching or rounding of the lower back.
   - If you feel any strain in your lower back, adjust the height of your hips or decrease the range of motion of your leg movements.
   - Aim to perform the exercise with smooth, fluid movements, rather than jerky or rushed motions.
   - Start with a small number of repetitions and gradually increase as you build strength and stability.

6. Variations:
   - To increase the challenge, you can hold a light resistance band around your thighs or ankles while performing the wall marches.
   - You can also add a pause at the bottom of each march, holding your foot just above the floor for a few seconds before lifting it back up.
   - For a greater challenge to your balance and stability, you can perform the wall marches on a stability ball instead of the floor.

Tips for Wall Marches:

- Maintain proper posture by keeping your back straight, shoulders relaxed, and avoiding overarching or rounding of the spine.

- Focus on engaging the core muscles throughout the exercise to stabilize the movement.

- Perform the exercise in a controlled manner, avoiding rapid or jerky movements.

Benefits of Wall Marches:

- Core Activation: Engages the core muscles, particularly the lower abdominals, to improve stability and balance.

- Hip Flexor Activation: Activates the hip flexor muscles, aiding in improving flexibility and range of motion in the hips.

- Balance Improvement: Enhances balance and coordination, especially when performed with focus on stability.

40. The Spine Stretch

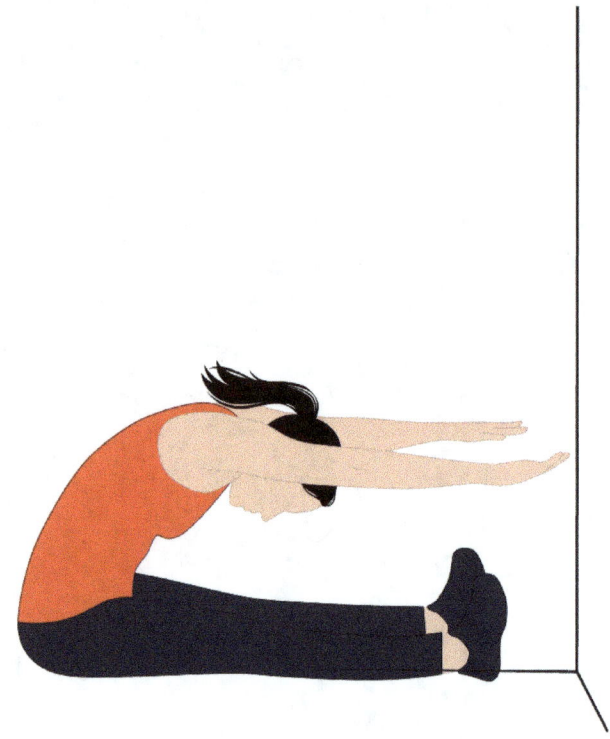

How to do the Spine Stretch:

1. Starting Position:

   o Sit tall on the floor or on an exercise mat with your legs extended straight in front of you.

   o Keep your feet flexed, legs together, and arms reaching forward at shoulder height.

2. Engage Core Muscles: engage your core by drawing your navel toward your spine to maintain stability throughout the exercise.

3. Performing the Movement:

   o Inhale to prepare. As you exhale, begin to articulate your spine by initiating the movement from the lower back.

   o Imagine each vertebrae peeling off the mat or floor one at a time as you start to round your spine forward.

4. Reach Forward:

- o Continue rounding forward, reaching your arms forward, and try to bring your head towards your knees or shins.

- o Avoid forcing yourself into the stretch; go only as far as your flexibility allows while maintaining a gentle stretch.

5. Hold and Breathe: hold the stretch for a few seconds while breathing deeply and relaxing into the position.

6. Return to Starting Position: inhale and slowly begin to stack your spine back up, vertebra by vertebra, starting from the lower back, until you are sitting tall again.

7. Repetition: repeat the movement, articulating your spine as you exhale and round forward, then returning to the starting position as you inhale.

Tips for the Spine Stretch:

- Focus on maintaining a smooth and controlled movement throughout without jerking or straining.

- Keep your shoulders relaxed and away from your ears during the exercise.

- Avoid locking your knees; keep them slightly bent throughout the movement.

Benefits of the Spine Stretch:

- Spine Flexibility: Stretches and mobilizes the entire length of the spine, promoting spinal flexibility and mobility.

- Improved Posture: Helps in elongating the spine and promotes better posture.

- Core Engagement: Engages the core muscles, especially during the return to the starting position, strengthening the core.

41. Wall Frog Stretch

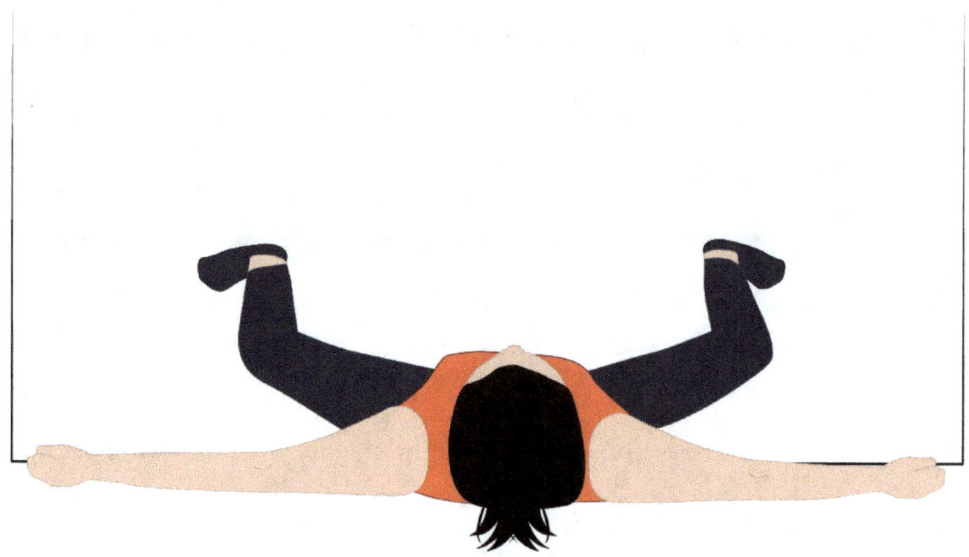

How to do the Wall Frog Stretch:

1. Starting Position:

    o   Lie on your back on an exercise mat or the floor near a wall.

    o   Position yourself close to the wall and extend your legs vertically, resting your feet against the wall.

    o   Your buttocks should be as close to the wall as comfortable, and your legs should be in an L-shape against the wall.

2. Opening the Legs:

    o   Open your legs into a wide position, allowing gravity to gently bring your legs towards the sides.

    o   Keep your feet flexed and the soles of your feet facing the ceiling.

3. Relax and Hold:

    o   Once in the widest comfortable position, relax into the stretch and hold the stretch for about 20-30 seconds.

- Focus on breathing deeply and relaxing your muscles as you feel the stretch in your inner thighs and groins.

4. Increasing the Stretch (Optional):

- If you feel comfortable and want to deepen the stretch, gently press your knees or thighs towards the floor, keeping the movement slow and controlled.

- Go only as far as your flexibility allows without causing discomfort or pain.

5. Hold and Breathe: hold the stretch at a comfortable level and continue to breathe deeply and evenly throughout the stretch.

6. Returning to Starting Position: to release the stretch, engage your inner thigh muscles and slowly bring your legs together, returning to the starting position with your feet against the wall.

Tips for Wall Frog Stretch:

- Focus on relaxing into the stretch rather than forcing your legs apart.

- Avoid bouncing or jerking movements; instead, perform the stretch smoothly and gradually.

- Listen to your body and stop if you feel any sharp pain.

Benefits of the Wall Frog Stretch:

- Inner Thigh Flexibility: Helps increase flexibility in the inner thighs (adductors) and groin area.

- Hip Mobility: Improves hip mobility and range of motion.

- Relaxation: Can promote relaxation and reduce tension in the hip and groin muscles.

42. Wall Pec Stretch

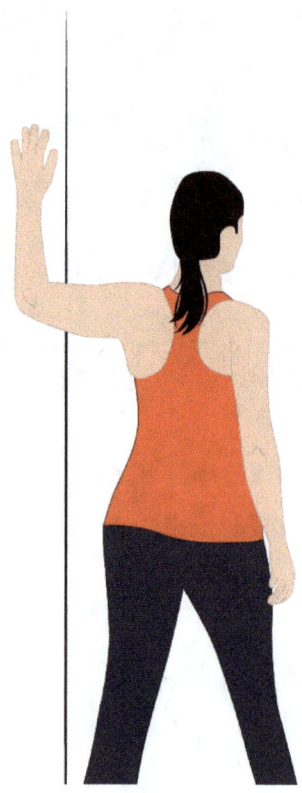

How to do the Wall Pec Stretch:

1. Starting Position:

   o   Stand facing a wall or a doorway.

   o   Extend your arm to the side and place your forearm against the wall, keeping your elbow at shoulder height. Your arm should be bent at a 90-degree angle.

2. Positioning the Body: take a small step forward with the foot on the same side as the arm against the wall. Your body will start to rotate away from the wall.

3. Engage the Stretch:

   o   Lean your body forward slightly until you feel a gentle stretch across the front of your chest and shoulder of the extended arm.

   o   You should feel a stretch along the pectoral muscles.

4. Hold the Stretch:

   o   Hold the stretch for about 20-30 seconds, while breathing deeply and relaxing into the stretch.

- Focus on maintaining a comfortable stretch without any pain or discomfort.

5. Switching Sides: release the stretch and switch to stretch the opposite side by repeating the same steps with your other arm.

Tips for the Wall Pec Stretch:

- Ensure your arm is bent at a 90-degree angle against the wall to target the chest muscles effectively.

- Maintain a relaxed posture and avoid arching your back excessively during the stretch.

- Keep your movements smooth and controlled, and avoid bouncing or forcing the stretch.

Benefits of the Wall Pec Stretch:

- Chest Flexibility: Helps in stretching and releasing tension in the chest muscles, particularly the pectoral muscles.

- Shoulder Mobility: Aids in improving shoulder flexibility and range of motion.

- Posture Support: Regular stretching of the chest muscles can contribute to better posture by counteracting rounded shoulders.

43. The Control Balance

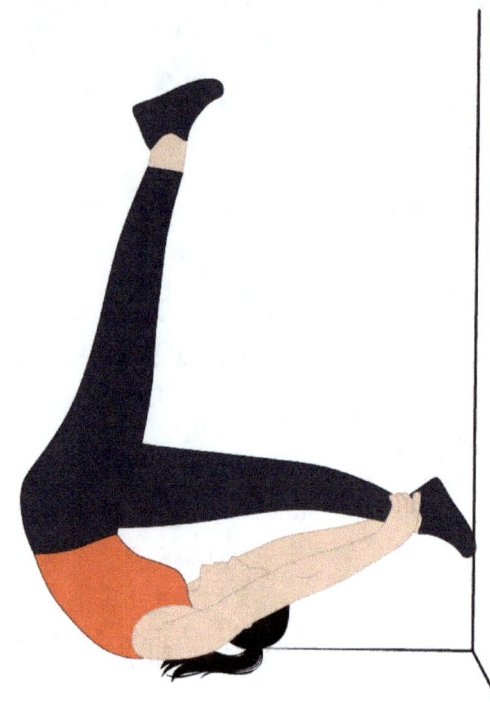

How to do a Modified Control Balance (Mat Version):

1. Starting Position: begin by lying flat on your back on an exercise mat with your arms alongside your body.

2. Leg Position:

    o Lift your legs off the mat, bend your knees, and bring them towards your chest.

    o Extend your legs towards the ceiling, aiming to create a tabletop position with your legs perpendicular to the floor.

3. Lifting into Balance:

    o Exhale and engage your core muscles deeply.

    o Using your abdominal strength, begin to lift your hips and lower back off the mat, aiming to balance on your tailbone while keeping your legs extended upwards.

4. Balancing Act:

    o Try to straighten your legs as much as possible, keeping them parallel to the floor. Your body will form a "V" shape, balancing on your tailbone and upper buttocks.

- Extend your arms alongside your legs or hold onto the back of your thighs for support.

5. Maintaining Balance:
   - Focus on stability and balance, engaging your core, and finding control in the lifted position.
   - Hold the balance for a few seconds while breathing steadily.

6. Returning to Starting Position: slowly lower your body back down with control, returning to the starting position on your back with legs extended towards the ceiling.

Tips for Modified Control Balance:

- This exercise requires considerable core strength and balance. Start by attempting it with caution and avoid overexertion.

- Engage your abdominal muscles throughout the movement to support your lower back.

- Avoid straining your neck or shoulders; focus on using your core muscles to lift and control the movement.

Benefits of the Control Balance:

- Core Strength: Engages and strengthens the core muscles, including the abdominals and obliques.

- Balance and Control: Improves balance, stability, and control over the body in a challenging position.

- Full-Body Engagement: Activates multiple muscle groups simultaneously, including the abdominals, hip flexors, and leg muscles.

44. Downward Facing Dog

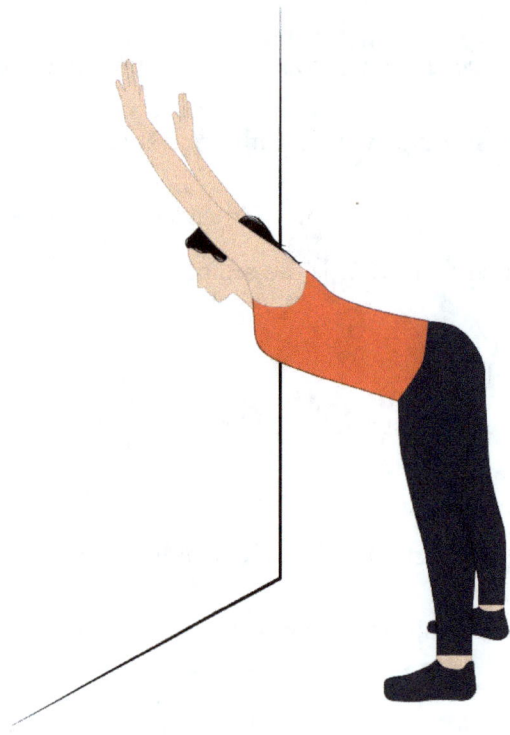

How to do Downward Facing Dog:

1. Setup:

    o   Stand facing a wall with your feet hip-width apart.

    o   Place your hands on the wall slightly above shoulder height, about shoulder-width apart.

    o   Your fingers should be spread wide, with your middle fingers pointing directly forward.

    o   Step back with your feet, allowing your body to hinge at the hips and create an inverted "V" shape.

2. Alignment:

    o   Press your palms firmly into the wall, distributing the weight evenly across your hands.

    o   Engage your core muscles to support your lower back and pelvis.

    o   Straighten your arms and legs as much as possible without locking your elbows or knees.

    o   Relax your neck and let your head hang between your arms, allowing it to align with your upper arms or gaze towards your navel.

3. Positioning:

- Press through your palms and actively push your hips upward and backward, creating length through your spine.
- Aim to bring your chest closer to your thighs while maintaining the length in your spine.
- Keep your heels grounded on the floor. They may not touch the floor completely, especially if you have tight hamstrings, but work towards bringing them down.

4. Breathing:

- Take slow, deep breaths in and out through your nose.
- Inhale as you lengthen through your spine and exhale as you deepen into the stretch.

5. Stretching:

- Feel the stretch along the back of your legs (hamstrings and calves), as well as your shoulders, arms, and upper back.
- If you feel any discomfort in your wrists, you can adjust the angle of your hands slightly or try pressing more through the base of your fingers.

6. Hold:

- Hold the pose for 30 seconds to 1 minute, breathing deeply and maintaining awareness of your alignment.
- If you're using this as a warm-up or part of a flow, you can hold it for shorter durations.

7. Release:

- To release the pose, gently walk your feet forward towards the wall until you're standing upright again.
- Shake out your arms and legs to release any tension.

8. Repeat: You can repeat the Downward Facing Dog on the wall a few times, focusing on your breath and alignment with each repetition.

Tips for Downward Facing Dog:

- It's okay if your heels don't touch the ground initially; focus on lengthening the spine and pressing through the palms.

- Engage your core muscles to support your lower back and maintain stability in the pose.

- Modify the pose by bending your knees slightly if you feel excessive strain in your hamstrings or lower back.

Benefits of Downward Facing Dog:

- Stretches and Strengthens: Provides a deep stretch for the entire body, especially the shoulders, hamstrings, calves, and spine.

- Improves Posture: Helps in elongating the spine and improving overall posture.

- Relaxation and Calming: Known for its calming effect on the mind and relieving stress.

45. Wall Wrist Stretches

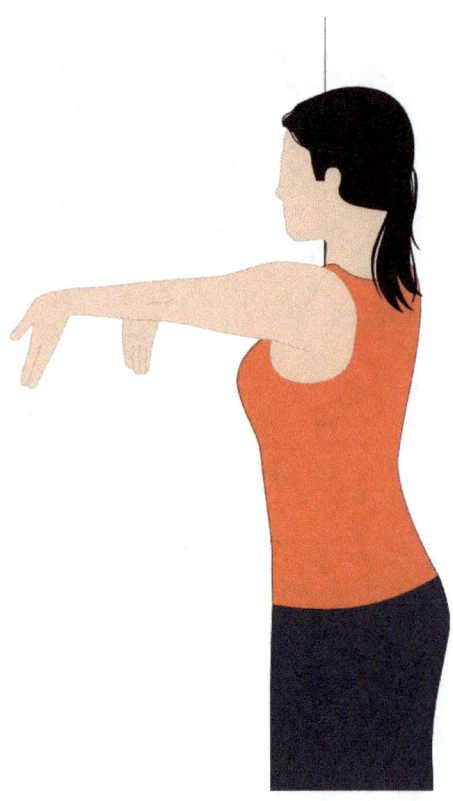

Wrist Flexor Stretch:

1. Facing the Wall:

    o Stand facing a wall and extend your arm straight in front of you, at shoulder height.

    o Place your palm against the wall, fingers pointing down, with your fingers spread apart.

2. Stretching the Wrist:

    o Keeping your arm straight, gently lean your body forward, allowing your palm to stay in contact with the wall.

    o You'll feel a stretch along the underside of your wrist and forearm.

3. Hold and Breathe:

    o Hold the stretch for about 15-30 seconds while maintaining a gentle, steady stretch.

    o Breathe deeply and relax into the stretch.

4. Switch Sides: release the stretch and switch to the other arm, repeating the same steps.

Wrist Extensor Stretch:

1. Positioning Against the Wall:

    - Stand facing away from the wall and extend your arm straight behind you, at shoulder height.

    - Place the back of your hand against the wall, fingers pointing down, with your fingers spread apart.

2. Stretching the Wrist Extensors:

    - Gently lean your body forward, maintaining the contact of the back of your hand against the wall.

    - You'll feel a stretch along the top of your wrist and forearm.

3. Hold and Relax: hold the stretch for about 15-30 seconds, breathing steadily and allowing the stretch to relax your wrist.

4. Switch Sides: release the stretch and repeat the same steps with the other arm.

Tips for Wall Wrist Stretches:

- Ensure the stretches are gentle and avoid forcing the wrists into uncomfortable positions.

- Keep your movements controlled and maintain a relaxed breathing pattern throughout the stretches.

- If you have any existing wrist injuries or conditions, consult a healthcare professional before performing these stretches.

Benefits of Wall Wrist Stretches:

- Flexibility Improvement: Helps increase flexibility and mobility in the wrist and forearm muscles.

- Relaxation and Tension Release: Relieves tension and stiffness commonly experienced in the wrists from repetitive movements or typing.

- Preventive Care: Regular stretching can aid in preventing wrist-related issues and conditions.

46. Wall Butterfly Stretch

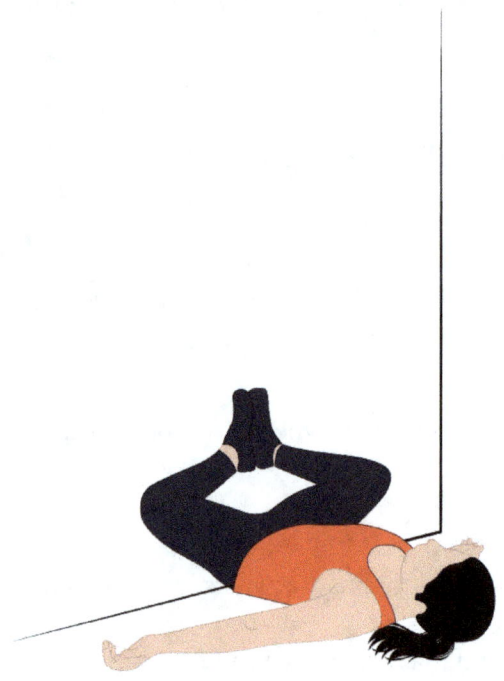

How to do the Wall Butterfly Stretch:

1. Setup:

- Lie on your back on the floor with your buttocks close to a wall.

- Extend your legs straight up against the wall, forming a 90-degree angle with your body.

- Your legs should be relaxed, with your feet flexed and your heels touching the wall.

- Allow your arms to rest comfortably by your sides.

2. Butterfly Position:

- Open your knees out to the sides, bringing the soles of your feet together.

- Allow your knees to bend naturally, creating a diamond shape with your legs.

- Your legs should resemble the wings of a butterfly, with your knees dropping towards the floor and your feet coming close to your groin.

3. Positioning:

- Adjust the distance between your buttocks and the wall to find a comfortable stretch in your inner thighs and groin area.
- Your feet should be in contact with each other, with the soles facing upward and the heels resting against the wall.
- Your arms can remain relaxed by your sides or placed in any comfortable position that helps you maintain balance and relaxation.

4. Relaxation and Breathing:

- Relax into the stretch, allowing the weight of your legs to gently open your hips.
- Take slow, deep breaths, inhaling through your nose and exhaling through your mouth.
- With each exhale, try to release any tension in your muscles and sink deeper into the stretch.

5. Duration:

- Hold the stretch for 30 seconds to 2 minutes, depending on your comfort level and flexibility.
- You can gradually increase the duration as you become more accustomed to the stretch.

6. Release:

- To release the stretch, gently bring your knees together, using your hands to assist if needed.
- Straighten your legs and rest them flat against the wall for a moment to allow your muscles to relax.

7. Repeat:

- You can repeat the Wall Butterfly Stretch multiple times, allowing your muscles to relax and lengthen with each repetition.
- Be mindful not to overstretch, and listen to your body's signals to avoid discomfort or strain.

Tips for Wall Butterfly Stretch:

- Find a position against the wall where your knees can comfortably open without causing discomfort.

- Avoid forcing your knees towards the ground; let gravity assist in the stretch gradually.

- Perform this stretch gently, especially if you have any existing groin or hip injuries.

Benefits of the Wall Butterfly Stretch:

- Inner Thigh Flexibility: Stretches and increases flexibility in the inner thighs and groin area.

- Relaxation: Helps in releasing tension and tightness in the groin muscles.

- Improved Range of Motion: Regular practice can enhance flexibility and improve the range of motion in the hip joints.

47. High Lunge Pose

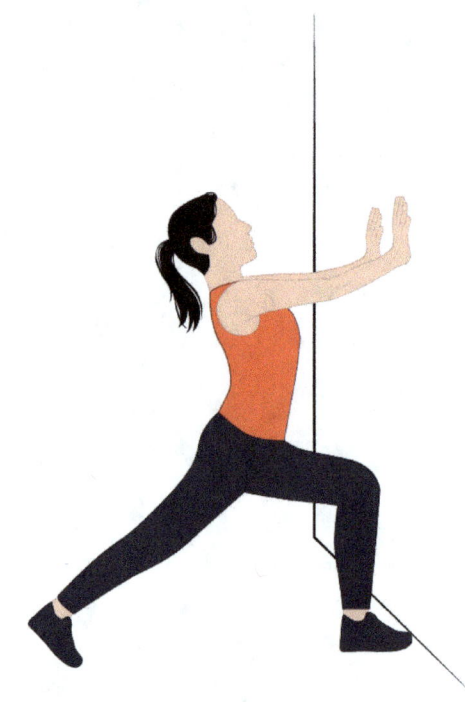

How to do High Lunge Pose:

1. Starting Position: begin in a standing position at the top of your yoga mat (or any comfortable surface).

2. Step Back: take a step back with your right foot, extending it behind you while keeping the ball of your foot on the ground and the heel lifted.

3. Lunge Position: bend your left knee, ensuring it is stacked directly above your left ankle. Your left thigh should be parallel to the floor, forming a lunge position.

4. Leg Alignment: your back leg (right leg) should be extended behind you with your knee straight, actively pressing the heel back.

5. Upper Body Position:

    o   Lift your torso upright and engage your core muscles to support your spine.

    o   Keep your shoulders relaxed and away from your ears.

6. Arms: extend your arms upward toward the ceiling, palms facing each other. Your arms should be in line with your ears.

7. Gaze and Breathing:

    - Soften your gaze forward or slightly upward.

    - Take deep and steady breaths, maintaining focus and balance.

8. Hold the Pose: hold the High Lunge Pose for about 30 seconds to 1 minute or longer if comfortable, maintaining proper alignment and breathing rhythm.

9. Release the Pose:

    - To release, gently lower your right knee to the ground and step forward to return to a standing position.

    - Repeat the pose by switching sides, stepping your left foot back this time.

Tips for High Lunge Pose:

- Ensure your front knee remains aligned with your ankle, avoiding it to extend past the ankle to protect the knee joint.

- Engage your core muscles to maintain stability and balance.

- You can modify the pose by placing your hands on your hips or keeping your hands in a prayer position at your chest for balance.

Benefits of High Lunge Pose:

- Lower Body Strengthening: Strengthens the legs, particularly the quadriceps and glutes.

- Hip Flexor Stretch: Stretches and opens the hip flexors.

- Balance and Focus: Enhances balance, stability, and concentration.

48. Wall Roll Downs

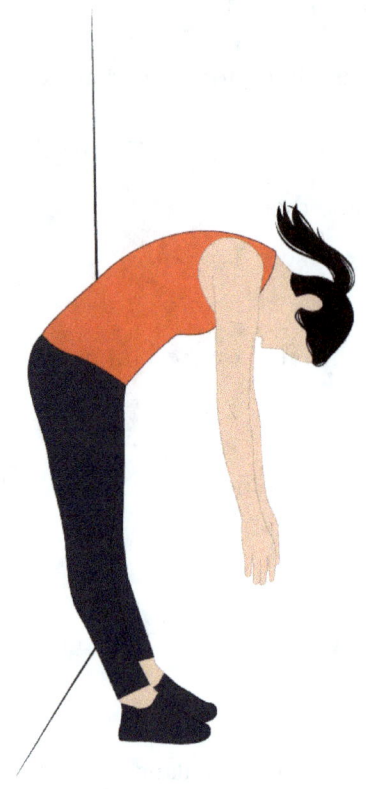

How to do Wall Roll-Downs:

1. Starting Position:

    - Stand with your back against a wall, feet hip-width apart, and a slight distance away from the wall.

    - Ensure your head, upper back, and hips are in contact with the wall.

2. Engage Core Muscles: engage your abdominal muscles by gently drawing your navel towards your spine.

3. Chin Tuck: begin the movement by gently tucking your chin towards your chest to lengthen the back of your neck.

4. Articulating the Spine: slowly start to roll down through your spine, one vertebra at a time, without forcefully arching your lower back.

5. Moving Downward:

    - Lower your chin towards your chest and start to round your upper back, allowing your mid-back, then lower back to peel away from the wall.

    - Keep your knees slightly bent throughout the movement to ease any tension in the hamstrings.

6. Stretch and Breathe:

- Continue rolling down until your arms hang naturally towards the floor or until you feel a comfortable stretch along your spine and the back of your legs.
- Take deep breaths while maintaining the stretched position for a few moments.

7. Reversing the Movement:

- Slowly reverse the movement by articulating your spine back up, starting from the lower back, then the mid-back, and finally the upper back.
- Aim to return to the standing position with your back, head, and hips aligned against the wall.

Tips for Wall Roll-Downs:

- Perform the movement slowly and mindfully, focusing on each vertebra's movement.

- Keep your shoulders relaxed and avoid tensing your neck or jaw during the exercise.

- Do not force the stretch; go only as far as your flexibility allows without discomfort.

Benefits of Wall Roll-Downs:

- Spinal Mobility: Enhances flexibility and mobility throughout the spine, promoting better movement and posture.

- Stretching: Stretches the back muscles, hamstrings, and helps release tension in the upper body.

- Posture Improvement: Encourages better alignment and awareness of spinal positioning.

48. Warrior 3 Pose

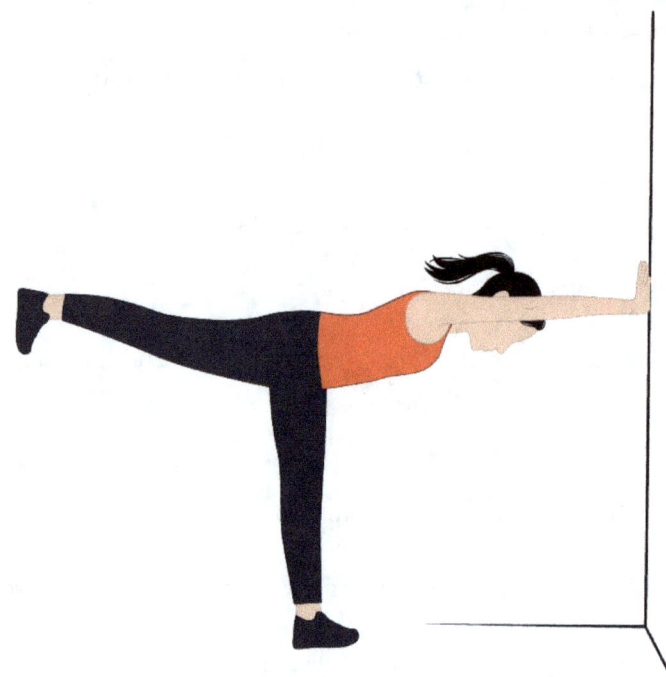

How to do Warrior 3 Pose:

1. Starting Position: begin in the Mountain Pose (Tadasana) at the top of your mat with your feet hip-width apart, arms by your sides.

2. Transition to Warrior 3: shift your weight onto your right foot and slightly lift your left foot off the ground, keeping your toes on the mat for balance.

3. Hinge Forward:

   - Hinge forward from your hips, extending your left leg straight back behind you while simultaneously lowering your torso towards the floor.

   - Your body should create a "T" shape, with your extended left leg, torso, and arms forming a straight line parallel to the floor.

4. Arms and Torso Position: Reach your arms forward alongside your ears, palms facing each other, or keep your hands in a prayer position at your chest for balance.

5. Alignment and Balance:

- Ensure your left leg and torso are in one straight line, parallel to the floor, forming a straight line from your head to your extended heel.
- Engage your core muscles to maintain balance and stability.

6. Focus and Breathing:
    - Gaze at a point on the floor ahead of you to assist with balance. Keep your neck in a neutral position.
    - Take slow and steady breaths, maintaining focus and control.

7. Hold the Pose: hold the Warrior 3 Pose for about 20-30 seconds or longer if comfortable, maintaining proper alignment and steady breathing.

8. Release the Pose:
    - To release, slowly lower your extended left leg to the floor and return to the Mountain Pose.
    - Repeat the pose on the other side by shifting your weight to the left foot and extending the right leg behind you.

Tips for Warrior 3 Pose:

- Keep your hips squared and facing towards the ground to maintain proper alignment.

- Engage your core muscles and avoid arching or rounding your back excessively.

- Start with shorter holds and gradually increase the duration as you build strength and balance.

Benefits of Warrior 3 Pose:

- Leg Strength: Strengthens the legs, particularly the quadriceps, hamstrings, and ankles.

- Balance and Stability: Improves balance, coordination, and stability.

- Focus and Concentration: Enhances mental focus and concentration by requiring full-body awareness.

50. Half Plough Pose

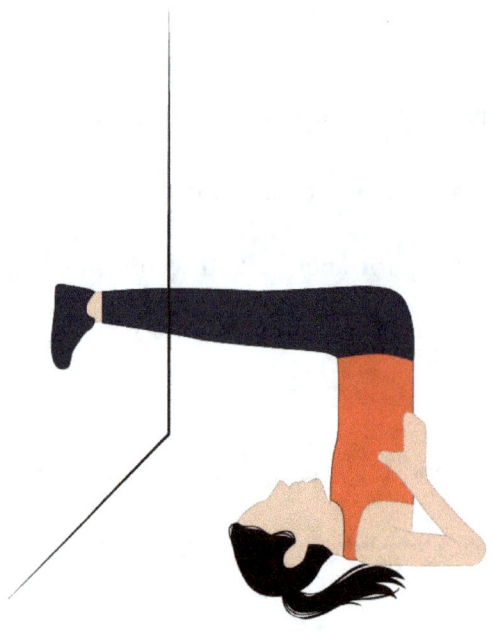

How to do Half Plough Pose:

1. Starting Position: begin by lying flat on your back on an exercise mat or the floor, with your legs extended and arms resting alongside your body, palms facing down.

2. Legs Position: inhale and lift your legs towards the ceiling, keeping them straight. If possible, hold the back of your right thigh with both hands for support.

3. Lowering the Legs:

    - Exhale and slowly lower your legs towards the wall behind your head.

    - Only lower the legs as far as is comfortable; it's not necessary for the toes to touch the wall.

4. Supporting the Back: use your hands to support your lower back or hips if needed, providing gentle support as you lower the legs.

5. Alignment and Breathing:

    - Ensure that your neck and head remain relaxed on the mat, avoiding strain or discomfort.

    - Maintain slow and steady breathing throughout the pose.

6. Hold the Pose: hold the Half Plough Pose for about 20-30 seconds, feeling a stretch along the back of your legs and the spine.

7. Return to Starting Position:

- To release the pose, engage your core muscles and slowly bring your legs back up towards the ceiling.
- Lower your legs to the floor, returning to the starting position with both legs extended.

Tips for Half Plough Pose:

- Ensure that you maintain control throughout the movement and avoid any sudden or jerky motions.

- Focus on lengthening the back of your leg and spine while performing the pose.

- Do not force your leg to lower too far if it causes discomfort or strain.

Benefits of Half Plough Pose:

- Spinal Stretch: Stretches and elongates the spine, promoting flexibility in the back.

- Hamstring and Calf Stretch: Helps in stretching the hamstrings and calves, aiding flexibility in the legs.

- Relaxation: Can have a calming effect on the body and mind when performed mindfully and with controlled breathing.

Chapter 3: 21-Day Transformation Challenge

Introduction to the 21-Day Challenge

Welcome to the transformative journey of Wall Pilates workouts! In the next 21 days, you are embarking on a dedicated path to enhance your physical strength, flexibility, and overall well-being. This challenge is designed to introduce you to a series of invigorating exercises aimed at utilizing the power of Pilates against the support of a wall.

The Wall Pilates Challenge is not just about workouts; it's a holistic approach towards achieving your fitness goals. Each day, you'll delve into a range of exercises carefully curated to engage your core, improve balance, and enhance flexibility. Whether you're a beginner or someone familiar with Pilates, this challenge caters to all levels, ensuring a gradual progression throughout the journey.

Through consistent dedication and perseverance, you'll witness the incredible benefits of these exercises, not only in your physical body but also in your mental focus and emotional well-being. As you commit yourself to these daily workouts, remember that every effort counts and brings you closer to the best version of yourself.

This guide will provide you with a structured program, comprising 50 diverse Wall Pilates exercises, specifically curated for women seeking a transformative fitness experience. Alongside the exercises, you'll find detailed instructions, tips for correct form, and modifications to suit individual needs.

Get ready to revitalize your body, rejuvenate your mind, and embrace the rewarding journey ahead. Let's embark together on this 21-day challenge and witness the incredible changes that await you!

Are you ready to unleash the power of Wall Pilates and transform yourself in just 21 days? Let's get started!

Daily Schedule and Workout Plan

Day 1:

- Warm-up: Wall Marches (3 sets of 15 reps)

- Main Workout: Wall Plank (3 sets of 30 seconds hold)

- Cool-down: Wall Pec Stretch (Hold for 30 seconds each side)

Day 2:

- Warm-up: Wall Marches (3 sets of 15 reps)

- Main Workout: Wall Squats (3 sets of 12 reps)

- Cool-down: Standing Glute Kickbacks (3 sets of 10 reps each leg)

Day 3:

- Warm-up: Wall Marches (3 sets of 15 reps)

- Main Workout: Wall Push-Ups (3 sets of 12 reps)

- Cool-down: Wall Hip Flexor Stretches (Hold for 30 seconds each side)

Day 4:

- Warm-up: Wall Marches (3 sets of 15 reps)

- Main Workout: Wall Sit with Leg Lifts (3 sets of 10 reps each leg)

- Cool-down: Wall Dead Bug (3 sets of 10 reps each side)

Day 5:

- Warm-up: Wall Marches (3 sets of 15 reps)

- Main Workout: Wall Bridge (3 sets of 15 reps)

- Cool-down: Wall Side Leg Lifts (3 sets of 12 reps each leg)

Day 6:

- Warm-up: Wall Marches (3 sets of 15 reps)

- Main Workout: Wall Sit (Hold for 1 minute)

- Cool-down: Wall Figure 4 Stretch (Hold for 30 seconds each side)

Day 7:

- Rest day or light stretching and mobility exercises.

Day 8:

- Warm-up: Wall Marches (3 sets of 15 reps)

- Main Workout: Seated Side Bends (3 sets of 12 reps each side)

- Cool-down: Wall Shoulder Taps (3 sets of 15 taps each side)

Day 9:

- Warm-up: Wall Marches (3 sets of 15 reps)

- Main Workout: Wall Calf Raises (3 sets of 20 reps)

- Cool-down: Legs Up the Wall (Hold for 1 minute)

Day 10:

- Warm-up: Wall Marches (3 sets of 15 reps)

- Main Workout: Wall Side Plank (Hold for 30 seconds each side)

- Cool-down: Wall Hamstring Stretches (Hold for 30 seconds each side)

Day 11:

- Warm-up: Wall Marches (3 sets of 15 reps)

- Main Workout: Wall Donkey Kicks (3 sets of 15 reps each leg)

- Cool-down: Wall Push-Ups with Leg Lifts (3 sets of 10 reps each leg)

Day 12:

- Warm-up: Wall Marches (3 sets of 15 reps)

- Main Workout: Wall Bicycle Crunches (3 sets of 15 reps each side)

- Cool-down: Wall Side Leg Lifts (3 sets of 12 reps each leg)

Day 13:

- Warm-up: Wall Marches (3 sets of 15 reps)

- Main Workout: Wall Crunches (3 sets of 15 reps)

- Cool-down: Wall Russian Twists (3 sets of 15 reps each side)

Day 14:

- Rest day or light stretching and mobility exercises.

Day 15:

- Warm-up: Wall Marches (3 sets of 15 reps)

- Main Workout: Wall Arm Circles (3 sets of 20 reps)

- Cool-down: Wall Angel (3 sets of 12 reps)

Day 16:

- Warm-up: Wall Marches (3 sets of 15 reps)

- Main Workout: Standing Glute Kickbacks (3 sets of 12 reps each leg)

- Cool-down: Wall Figure 4 Stretch (Hold for 30 seconds each side)

Day 17:

- Warm-up: Wall Marches (3 sets of 15 reps)

- Main Workout: Wall Dead Bug (3 sets of 12 reps each side)

- Cool-down: Wall Hip Flexor Stretches (Hold for 30 seconds each side)

Day 18:

- Warm-up: Wall Marches (3 sets of 15 reps)

- Main Workout: Standing Wall Twist (3 sets of 15 reps each side)

- Cool-down: Wall Side Lunges (3 sets of 12 reps each side)

Day 19:

- Warm-up: Wall Marches (3 sets of 15 reps)

- Main Workout: Wall Walks (3 sets of 5 walks)

- Cool-down: Wall Sprints (high knees against the wall) (3 sets of 20 seconds)

Day 20:

- Warm-up: Wall Marches (3 sets of 15 reps)

- Main Workout: Wall Splits (Hold for 30 seconds)

- Cool-down: Wall Tricep Stretch (Hold for 30 seconds each side)

Day 21:

- Warm-up: Wall Marches (3 sets of 15 reps)

- Main Workout: Wall Squats (3 sets of 15 reps)

- Cool-down: The Spine Stretch (Hold for 30 seconds)

This comprehensive 21-day workout plan integrates various exercises targeting different muscle groups, balance, and flexibility. Always ensure proper form and technique during exercises, and listen to your body for any signs of fatigue or discomfort.

Consistency and dedication to this plan, coupled with a balanced diet and adequate rest, will help maximize the benefits of the Wall Pilates workouts and contribute to your overall fitness journey. Adjust the plan according to your fitness level and personal preferences to achieve the best results while avoiding strain or overexertion.

Chapter 4: Nutrition and Wellness

21-Day Meal Plan

Day 1:

Breakfast: Greek yogurt with berries and almonds

Lunch: Grilled chicken salad with mixed greens, cherry tomatoes, cucumbers, and vinaigrette

Dinner: Baked salmon with quinoa and steamed vegetables

Day 2:

Breakfast: Oatmeal topped with sliced bananas and a sprinkle of chia seeds

Lunch: Whole-grain wrap with hummus, mixed veggies, and grilled tofu

Dinner: Turkey chili with kidney beans and a side of roasted sweet potatoes

Day 3:

Breakfast: Spinach and feta omelet with whole-grain toast

Lunch: Quinoa salad with chickpeas, diced veggies, and lemon-tahini dressing

Dinner: Stir-fried tofu with broccoli, bell peppers, and brown rice

Day 4:

Breakfast: Smoothie with spinach, banana, almond milk, and protein powder

Lunch: Grilled shrimp with quinoa tabbouleh

Dinner: Baked chicken breast with roasted Brussels sprouts and sweet potato wedges

Day 5:

Breakfast: Whole-grain toast with avocado and poached eggs

Lunch: Lentil soup with a side of mixed greens salad

Dinner: Veggie stir-fry with tofu, served over cauliflower rice

Day 6:

Breakfast: Overnight oats with almond milk, berries, and a drizzle of honey

Lunch: Whole-grain pasta with marinara sauce, mixed veggies, and grilled chicken

Dinner: Baked cod with asparagus and quinoa pilaf

Day 7:

Breakfast: Whole-grain waffles topped with Greek yogurt and fresh fruit

Lunch: Tuna salad stuffed in bell peppers

Dinner: Turkey meatballs with zucchini noodles and marinara sauce

Day 8:

Breakfast: Chia seed pudding with mixed berries and a sprinkle of granola

Lunch: Grilled vegetable and quinoa salad with a lemon-herb vinaigrette

Dinner: Baked tofu with roasted root vegetables and a side of wild rice

Day 9:

Breakfast: Whole-grain toast with almond butter and sliced strawberries

Lunch: Black bean and corn salad with diced avocado and lime-cilantro dressing

Dinner: Grilled lemon-herb chicken breast with steamed broccoli and quinoa

Day 10:

Breakfast: Veggie omelet with bell peppers, onions, spinach, and a side of whole-grain toast

Lunch: Lentil curry with brown rice

Dinner: Baked cod with a side of sautéed kale and sweet potato mash

Day 11:

Breakfast: Smoothie bowl with mixed berries, spinach, almond milk, and a sprinkle of nuts and seeds

Lunch: Whole-grain wrap with grilled veggies, hummus, and shredded chicken

Dinner: Turkey and vegetable kebabs with quinoa tabbouleh

Day 12:

Breakfast: Protein pancakes topped with sliced bananas and a drizzle of honey

Lunch: Quinoa salad with mixed greens, roasted vegetables, and a balsamic vinaigrette

Dinner: Baked salmon with roasted Brussels sprouts and quinoa pilaf

Day 13:

Breakfast: Greek yogurt parfait with granola and mixed berries

Lunch: Chickpea and vegetable stir-fry with brown rice

Dinner: Grilled chicken breast with asparagus and sweet potato wedges

Day 14:

Breakfast: Whole-grain bagel with cream cheese and smoked salmon

Lunch: Tofu and vegetable curry with a side of quinoa

Dinner: Turkey chili with kidney beans and a mixed greens salad

Day 15:

Breakfast: Overnight oats with almond milk, sliced peaches, and a sprinkle of cinnamon

Lunch: Grilled vegetable and quinoa salad with a tahini dressing

Dinner: Baked chicken thighs with roasted carrots and a side of whole-grain couscous

Day 16:

Breakfast: Whole-grain toast topped with mashed avocado, sliced tomatoes, and a poached egg

Lunch: Lentil soup with a side of mixed greens and a whole-grain roll

Dinner: Baked cod with roasted asparagus and quinoa

Day 17:

Breakfast: Smoothie with spinach, mango, banana, and almond milk

Lunch: Whole-grain wrap with hummus, mixed veggies, and grilled chicken

Dinner: Turkey meatballs with zucchini noodles and marinara sauce

Day 18:

Breakfast: Greek yogurt with honey, chopped walnuts, and mixed berries

Lunch: Quinoa salad with chickpeas, diced veggies, and lemon-tahini dressing

Dinner: Stir-fried tofu with broccoli, bell peppers, and brown rice

Day 19:

Breakfast: Veggie omelet with bell peppers, onions, spinach, and a side of whole-grain toast

Lunch: Grilled shrimp with quinoa tabbouleh

Dinner: Baked chicken breast with roasted Brussels sprouts and sweet potato wedges

Day 20:

Breakfast: Whole-grain waffles topped with Greek yogurt and fresh fruit

Lunch: Tuna salad stuffed in bell peppers

Dinner: Veggie stir-fry with tofu, served over cauliflower rice

Day 21:

Breakfast: Chia seed pudding with mixed berries and a sprinkle of granola

Lunch: Lentil curry with brown rice

Dinner: Grilled lemon-herb chicken breast with steamed broccoli and quinoa

Don't forget to adjust portion sizes according to your individual needs and make any necessary modifications to suit your preferences or dietary requirements. Staying consistent with a well-rounded, nutritious meal plan will complement your Wall Pilates workouts and contribute to achieving your fitness goals. Enjoy the journey to a healthier you!

Mindfulness and Holistic Well-being

Incorporating mindfulness practices into your daily routine is integral to achieving holistic well-being during this 21-day Wall Pilates Challenge. Mindfulness isn't just about being present in the moment; it's a way of life that encourages awareness, self-compassion, and embracing the present journey.

As you engage in each Wall Pilates workout, invite mindfulness into your practice. Pay attention to your breath, the sensations in your body, and the connection between movement and mind. Embrace the present moment, acknowledging any thoughts or feelings that arise without judgment. This mindful awareness can amplify the benefits of your workouts, fostering a deeper mind-body connection.

Holistic well-being extends beyond physical fitness. It encompasses nurturing mental clarity, emotional stability, and spiritual alignment. The Wall Pilates Challenge isn't solely about sculpting the body; it's about fostering a sense of balance within yourself—physically, mentally, and emotionally.

Remember, well-being isn't achieved solely through exercise; it's a culmination of various factors—adequate rest, nourishing nutrition, mindful movement, emotional balance, and nurturing relationships. Throughout this journey, prioritize self-care, listen to your body's cues, and cultivate a supportive environment conducive to your growth.

Take moments to meditate, practice gratitude, and find joy in simple pleasures. Nurture your mind and spirit as much as you nurture your body. Embrace the transformative power of this challenge as a catalyst for holistic well-being—a journey that encompasses every facet of your being.

Let this 21-day challenge not only sculpt your body but also elevate your mind, uplift your spirit, and inspire a balanced, fulfilling lifestyle.

Conclusion

Congratulations on completing the 21-day Wall Pilates Challenge! You've reached a significant milestone in your journey towards a healthier, more balanced lifestyle. These past three weeks have been a testament to your commitment, perseverance, and dedication to your well-being.

Throughout this challenge, you've explored the transformative power of Wall Pilates—a journey that transcends mere physical exercise. You've delved into the realms of mindfulness, strength, and self-discovery. Each day, you stepped onto the mat, embracing the workouts with determination and openness.

Reflect on the progress you've made—celebrate the small victories and the strides you've taken towards a stronger, more flexible body. But beyond the physical changes, acknowledge the mental and emotional growth you've experienced. You've cultivated resilience, patience, and a deeper connection with yourself.

As you conclude this challenge, remember that this is just the beginning of your wellness journey. The habits and lessons learned during these 21 days will continue to shape your path forward. Carry forward the sense of empowerment and accomplishment you've gained.

The journey towards well-being extends far beyond these three weeks. It's about creating sustainable habits, nurturing self-care, and embracing a balanced lifestyle. Continue to honor your body, mind, and spirit by integrating movement, mindfulness, and self-compassion into your daily routine.

Take pride in how far you've come, and be excited about the possibilities that lie ahead. Let this challenge be a catalyst for ongoing growth, self-discovery, and the pursuit of a life filled with vitality and balance.

Thank you for dedicating yourself to this journey. May the strength, resilience, and mindfulness cultivated during these 21 days empower you to live a fulfilling and healthy life.

Continue to move forward, embrace every challenge, and thrive in your pursuit of wellness!